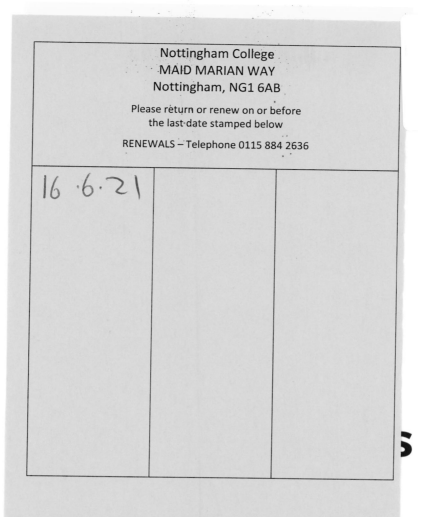
PRODUCED BY MATHSFORNURSES.COM

written by Tom O'Toole

Written by Tom O'Toole for MATHSFORNURSES.COM – www.mathsfornurses.com

Contents

Basic Numeracy Skills

Basic Numeracy Skills Practice Tests

Drug Calculation Skills

Drug Calculations Practice Tests

About Maths For Nurses

Why Maths for Nurses?

Nobody becomes a nurse to do Maths. If that's what you were into, you would have become an engineer, or an accountant, or a teacher.

You became a nurse because you want to help people.

But the truth is that numeracy skills are a vital part of what it means to be a nurse. In fact, the only Maths tests that I have ever come across where you need to score 100% to pass are the drug calculations tests that nurses are required to take.

Because of the nature of your work, you are expected to carry out mathematical calculations with unerring accuracy every day of your professional life.

For someone who didn't get into it to do Maths that's a big ask. Perhaps you could do with a bit of help?

That's where I come in.

I'm Tom. I am one of those people who wanted to get into Maths. I am a qualified Maths teacher and private tutor, and over the years, I have worked with quite a few nurses and nursing students who were struggling to get their head around the Maths that they needed to know for their drugs calculations tests.

It is this work that led me to write this book, create the www.mathsfornurses.com website and put together other resources to help. I knew that the lessons that I had taught in those one-on-one sessions could be invaluable for many others who find Maths a challenge and yet need it for their professional practice.

I am so glad you have got a copy of this book.

Let me just briefly mention a few other things that may be of interest to you.

Maths For Nurses Website

I have created the Maths for Nurses website as the online home of all things numeracy and nursing – please do take a good look around at www.mathsfornurses.com

Free Practice Tests

As well as the practice tests included in this book, I have created three more practice tests that are absolutely free. You can access them at www.mathsfornurses.com/free-practice-tests

Pass Your Drug Calculations Test with Ease

'Pass Your Drug Calculations Test with Ease' is an online course that I have created that is designed to turbo-charge your numeracy preparation. The course contains dozens of video tutorials, presenting every skill that you will need in easy-to-digest steps and demonstrating how to use the skills in real problems. Accompanying each video are cheat sheets and additional exercises for you to practice further, as well as access to support as you study to help you with any questions that you might have. Find out more at www.mathsfornurses.com/course

Coaching

Our bespoke coaching sessions are the ultimate in individualised support. After an initial consultation, you will get a one-on-one video call with me (Tom) and we will tailor the coaching around the particular areas of help that you need. After each coaching session, I will assign you further exercises to reinforce the things that you have learned on the call. Find out more at www.mathsfornurses.com/coaching

About Drug Calculations Tests

What Are Drug Calculations?

Drug calculations are a key part of the nursing profession.

When a patient has been given a prescription, it often falls to nurses to administer that prescription. It is of vital importance that the amount of drug administered is the same as that which was prescribed. This will usually require the nurse to perform calculations, as the final amount to administer may depend on the stock dose available, the drip rate of an infusion set, the weight of the patient, or one of many other factors.

What are Drug Calculations Tests?

To ensure that nurses are able to accurately perform the calculations that are required in their job, they will frequently be asked to take drug calculations tests, where they are presented with a set of hypothetical scenarios and asked to make calculations similar to those that their work would require.

Before starting a nursing course, aspiring nurses are expected to have attained a minimum of a grade C in their Maths GCSE, and will often be asked by their university to take a basic numeracy test before embarking on the course. These tests will focus on topics such as numerical calculations, fractions, decimals, percentages and converting between different units of measurement.

As the course goes on, further tests will be given, and these will usually shift the focus to using numeracy skills in the particular contexts that arise in the nursing profession, and a student will need to show their ability to make these calculations before they qualify.

Once qualified, nurses are given further drug calculations tests in many hospitals (sometimes annually) to ensure that their skills remain at the required level.

The precise tests vary between different hospitals and universities. There is no universally followed format for the tests, so make sure you find out from the test administrator the time limit, the number of questions, the style of questions, the difficulty level and whether or not a calculator is allowed for the test (they may be willing to give you some past papers to practice with).

Because of the high importance of performing drug calculations with accuracy, the pass rate for drug calculation tests is usually set at 100%.

About the Book

This book is designed to help you to develop the numeracy skills required for nursing. The book is in two parts (with 8 chapters in each). The first part focuses on basic numeracy methods, learning the skills without applying them to particular contexts. The second part of the book looks at applying these methods to the particular calculations that nurses are called upon to make.

In each chapter, there are 'Have a Go' questions that you can do to practice using the methods that have been taught, and at the end of the chapter is a further practice exercise made up of 10 more questions so that you can consolidate your skills.

After each part of the book, there are also some practice tests that you can try. There are four practice tests on the basic numeracy skills, and four on drug calculations.

The solutions to all practice questions are found at the end of the relevant chapters, and as a free bonus for readers of the book I have made available fully worked solutions for every question, showing you the methods that you could have used to get the correct answers. These solutions are available as free downloads at www.mathsfornurses.com and each chapter will contain the specific link on the site that you can use to get that set of worked solutions.

Paediatrics*

Whilst many of the skills overlap, there are some differences in the drug calculations carried out by nurses working with adults and nurses working in paediatrics. Topics indicated with a * contain material that is particularly relevant for paediatric nurses (this content may still be helpful for nurses who work with adults).

Ten Top Tips

1. Start with a Practice Test

Perhaps you have already seen the practice tests that are freely available at www.mathsfornurses.com/free-practice-tests

Doing these tests is a great start to your preparation as it will give you a feel for the kinds of questions you are likely to be asked and will help you see how close you are to being ready to sit the test.

Using these tests at this point means that you can save the tests that are in this book for later in your practice as a way of charting the progress that you make.

2. Identify Target Topics

Whilst there is value in refreshing your knowledge on all topics, it is essential to know which kinds of questions you consistently struggle with and to focus your revision on these areas.

3. Work on One Topic at Once

When you have identified a few topics that you want to focus on, it is helpful to tackle them one at a time. It is better to delve into one area until you are really confident in that subject before moving on to the next than to try to learn a little of everything at the same time, only to confuse yourself.

4. Try Practice Questions

Knowledge in Maths is not primarily gained by reading descriptions of principles and methods. These can be a helpful start, but to truly understand you will need to apply that knowledge to solving specific problems. Each chapter of this guide contains practice questions for you to work through, and there are fully worked solutions available for you to check your work.

5. Get the Basics Right

It is not unusual for people to approach a complicated question with the correct method and yet get the answer wrong because of a numerical error. Make sure that your methods for adding, subtracting, multiplying and dividing (including with decimals) are clear and accurate, and have instant recall of your times tables (at least up to 10 × 10 and ideally up to 12 × 12).

6. Be Clear what the Question Is Asking

Just because a question looks similar to one that you have done before doesn't mean that it is asking exactly the same thing. Make sure you read the questions carefully and are sure what they are asking you to do.

7. Check Your Answers

If you have time left at the end of the test, it is a good idea to use it to check your answers. This is also the case in the calculations in your professional practice. Check the answer a couple of times and if you are unsure which answer is correct, then consult with a pharmacist or the person who wrote the prescription (obviously this will not be an option when sitting the test!)

8. Kill Distractions

You will find it difficult to learn with the television on in the background and your smartphone next to your work. Put aside anything that will distract you and make sure the time you are giving to revision is entirely focussed on revising.

9. Start in the Right Frame of Mind

As tempting as it can be to pull an all-nighter cramming the night before the test, it is likely to be counter-productive. You will perform at your best when you are fresh and awake. Make sure you go into the test with a good night's sleep, good meals, and well hydrated, and give it your best shot.

10. Consider a Coaching Course

If you are still struggling with certain areas after working through practice papers and the methods suggested in this guide, then you may want to consider taking a course. There is a coaching course available at www.mathsfornurses.com/course that is called 'Pass Your Drug Calculations Test with Ease'. This course is a wonderful way to turbo-charge your preparation, and would be the natural next step if you want a bit more help.

Further Resources

For a free, up-to-date guide to different resources for drug calculations tests, please visit www.mathsfornurses.com/resources

Place Value

Numeracy is fundamentally about numbers, and as you build the numeracy skills required for nursing you will learn how to work with and manipulate numbers in different ways.

The starting point is by grasping how numbers work.

Numbers are made up of one or more digits, and each digit has a different value according to its place in the number (known as its 'place value').

For example, the number 342 has three digits, a '3' a '4' and a '2'.

The last of the digits is the 'units' digit (unless there is a decimal point in the number – see below). This means that the '2' is worth 2 ones, or just 2.

The next digit along (working from right to left) is the 'tens' digit. This means that the '4' is worth 4 tens, or 40.

The digit furthest left is the 'hundreds' digit. This means that the '3' is worth 3 hundreds, or 300.

The overall number is made up of 3 hundreds, 4 tens and 2 units.

If there were more digits before the hundreds, these would be thousands, ten-thousands, hundred-thousands and millions.

Have a Go

What is the value of each digit in the number 1769?

The Decimal Point

Often you will need to deal with numbers that are not exact. For example, the weight of a patient may not be exactly 42kg or 43kg but somewhere between the two.

You can express numbers like this by using a decimal point.

A decimal point is a dot written after the units digit, and more digits can be written after the decimal point.

For example, if you are told that the weight of a patient is 42.15kg, the decimal point is between the 2 and the 1.

The numbers before the decimal point tell you how many whole kilograms you have (read the number as above – 2 units and 4 tens is 42).

The numbers after the decimal point tell you that as well as the 42kg there is part of another kilogram.

Values of Digits After the Decimal Point

Just as each digit before the decimal point has a value determined by its place, so does each number after the decimal point.

For example, consider the number 42.15.

The first digit after the decimal point is the '1'. This digit tells you how many 'tenths' the number has (this means that if you split a whole unit into 10 pieces, how many of them would you have?). In this case, there is 1 tenth.

The second digit after the decimal point is the '5'. This digit tells you how many 'hundredths' the number has (this means that if you split a whole unit into 100 pieces, how many of them would you have?). In this case, there are 5 hundredths.

If there had been more digits after the decimal point, these would have been the 'thousandths', 'ten-thousandths', 'hundred-thousandths' and so on.

Have a Go

What is the value of each digit in the number 2.74?

Comparing Numbers

When you need to compare which of 2 numbers is largest, you can use the place value of the numbers to do so.

Start by comparing the digits worth the largest 'value' (if one of them does not have a digit in a certain place, treat it as having zero). For example, 1324 is larger than 867 because it has 1 thousand whereas 876 doesn't have any thousands.

The same principle applies to comparing decimal numbers. For example, if you need to compare 0.12 and 0.9, start by comparing the units digit in each number. As both are 0, move on to the next digit (the tenths). 0.12 has 1 tenth and 0.9 has 9 tenths so 0.9 is the larger number.

Have a Go

Which number is larger: 0.32 or 0.302?

You can use this same method to put a list of numbers in order. For example, if you need to order 9.65, 12.4, 9.06, 10.68 and 12.45.

A good tip to make this easier is to write the numbers in a column. If you ensure that the decimal points are directly beneath one another, then all of the digits will be lined up correctly according to their place value.

```
      9 . 6 5
   1  2 . 4
      9 . 0 6
   1  0 . 6 8
   1  2 . 4 5
```

Start by comparing the tens digits. 12.4, 10.68 and 12.45 have one ten each whereas the other numbers don't have any so these are the first three numbers.

Just for these three numbers, compare the units digits. 12.4 and 12.45 have 2 units each whereas 10.68 doesn't have any, so these are the largest two numbers and 10.68 is third.

Compare the tenths digits for these two numbers. They are both 4, so then compare the hundredths digits. 12.45 has 5 hundredths but 12.4 doesn't have any so 12.45 is the largest number and 12.4 is second.

Now work out which digits are fourth and fifth largest. The remaining two numbers are 9.65 and 9.06. They both have 9 units, but 9.65 has more tenths, so it is the fourth largest number and 9.06 is fifth largest.

From largest to smallest, the order of the numbers is 12.45, 12.4, 10.68, 9.65, 9.06.

Have a Go

Put these numbers in order from smallest to largest. 1.3, 0.31, 1.23, 0.1

Multiplying & Dividing by 10

You may have noticed that each digit in a number is worth 10 times more than the previous digit (a hundred is ten tens, a thousand is ten hundreds, etc.).

Because of this, if you multiply a number by ten, each digit in the number will 'move' one place to the left (the decimal point will remain unmoved).

For example, if you multiply 2.83 by 10, the 2 will move from 'units' to 'tens', the 8 will move from 'tenths' to 'units' and the 3 will move from 'hundredths' to 'tenths', so the answer will be 28.3

If moving the digits leaves a gap before the decimal point, fill the gap with a 0. For example 46 × 10 would turn the 4 into 'hundreds' and the 6 into 'tens' but leave a gap for the units, so you would write 0 units for an answer of 460.

Have a Go

Work out 35.61 × 10

In a similar way, when you divide a number by ten, each number will 'move' one place to the right.

For example, if you divide 17.2 by 10, the 1 will become 'units', the 7 will become 'tenths' and the 2 will become 'hundredths', giving an answer of 1.72.

Have a Go

Work out 35.61 ÷ 10

Multiplying & Dividing by Other Powers of 10

Multiplying a number by 100 is the same as multiplying a number by 10 and then by 10 again (because 100 is the same as 10 × 10). This means that to multiply a number by 100 you can move each digit two places to the left (and dividing by 100 would move each digit two places to the right).

For example, 18.94 × 100 would change the 1 from 'tens' to 'thousands' (moving one place would make it hundreds, so moving two places makes it thousands), the 8 from 'units' to 'hundreds', the 9 from 'tenths' to 'tens' and the 4 from 'hundredths' to 'units' meaning that the answer is 1894.

In a similar way, multiplying by 1000 would move the digits three places to the left and dividing by 1000 would move the digits three places to the right. The same principle can be applied to higher powers of 10 (if a number is a '1' followed by a string of zeroes, the number of zeroes is the same as the number of places that the digits need to be moved).

Calculations like this are very important when converting measurements from one unit to another (for example to convert a drug prescribed in milligrams into micrograms, you need to multiply the prescribed amount by 1000). This will be covered further in the chapter on 'Converting Measurements'.

Have a Go

Work out 255.4 ÷ 100

Have a Go

Work out 7.52 × 1000

Practice Questions

Question 1

What is the value of the 7 in 37846?

Question 2

What is the value of the 6 in 241.369?

Question 3

Which number is larger: 11.75 or 103.6?

Question 4

Which number is smaller: 0.037 or 0.324?

Question 5

Arrange these numbers in order from smallest to largest: 1.3, 1.303, 1.03, 1.33

Question 6

What is 362.1 × 10?

Question 7

What is 0.34 ÷ 10?

Question 8

What is 77.293 × 100?

Question 9

What is 211 ÷ 100?

Question 10

What is 0.03 × 1000?

Solutions

Fully worked solutions to all of these questions can be accessed at www.mathsfornurses.com/placevalue

Have a Go

1. 1 = 1000, 7 = 700, 6 = 60. 9 = 9

2. 2 = 2, 7 = $\frac{7}{10}$, 4 = $\frac{4}{100}$

3. 0.32

4. 0.1, 0.31, 1.23, 1.3

5. 356.1

6. 3.561

7. 2.554

8. 7520

Practice Questions

1. 7000

2. $\frac{6}{100}$

3. 103.6

4. 0.037

5. 1.03, 1.3, 1.303, 1.33

6. 3621

7. 0.034

8. 7729.3

9. 2.11

10. 30

Calculations

In order to perform drug calculations accurately, you need to have a good grasp of methods for adding, subtracting, multiplying and dividing numbers.

In your practice, you will often have access to a calculator to perform these calculations. However, it is important that you are confident in how to work out answers without the calculator for two reasons. Firstly, there may be situations where a calculator is not available to you, and secondly, you need to have an idea of the correct answer in order to have a sense of when a calculator gives an erroneous answer.

Addition

The basic building block of addition is adding together two single-digit numbers (e.g. 3 + 6 or 7 + 9). It makes the addition method a lot easier if you have the answers to all such calculations readily available for instant recall (though if you don't, you can work out the answers by 'counting on' the appropriate number of units).

When you are able to add single-digit numbers, you can use this to add larger numbers using the 'column method' of addition. Write the numbers that you want to add together above each other in columns, lined up according to their place value (i.e. the units digit of one number should be under the units digit of the other number, the tens digit under the tens digit and so on). If one of the numbers has more digits than another, this is okay – the space in that column for the other number will simply be left blank.

For example to work out 184 + 93, line up the numbers so that the 4 is above the 3 and the 8 is above the 9.

$$
\begin{array}{r}
1\ 8\ 4 \\
+\quad 9\ 3 \\
\hline
\\
\hline
\end{array}
$$

Starting with the units column and working from right to left, add together the numbers in each column and write the answer underneath. In this case, 4 + 3 = 7.

```
        1   8   4
    +       9   3
   _____
                    7
   _____
```

When you come on to the tens column, the answer is a two-digit number because 8 + 9 = 17. In this case, only write the units digit (the 7) as part of the answer and 'carry' the tens digit (the 1) into the next column to add together with the numbers in this column.

```
        1   8   4
    +   ₁   9   3
   _____
            7   7
   _____
```

In the hundreds column, there is the 1 from the top number, nothing from the second number and the 1 that has been carried. Add these together to get 1 + 1 = 2 and write this as the hundreds digit of the answer.

```
        1   8   4
    +   ₁   9   3
   _____
        2   7   7
   _____
```

The final answer is 277.

Have a Go

Work out 385 + 67

Adding Decimals

The same method can be used to add decimals. The important step is to ensure that the numbers are lined up by place value correctly (using the decimal points as a guide can be helpful). You may end up with blank columns in both numbers.

For example, if you need to work out 64.8 + 3.75, you would line up the numbers as below (notice that a decimal point has been written in the space for the answer, in a position that corresponds with the decimal points in the numbers that are being added together). Start by adding the numbers in the column on the right and work your way from right to left.

$$
\begin{array}{r}
6 \quad 4 \,.\, 8 \\
+ \quad 3 \,.\, 7 \quad 5 \\
\hline
. \\
\hline
\end{array}
$$

This can be added as before to get an answer of 68.55.

$$
\begin{array}{r}
6 \quad 4 \,.\, 8 \\
+ \quad 3 \,.\, 7 \quad 5 \\
\hline
\mathbf{6} \quad \mathbf{8} \,.\, \mathbf{5} \quad \mathbf{5} \\
\hline
\end{array}
$$

Have a Go

Work out 2.86 + 0.975

Subtraction

A column method can also be used for subtracting numbers. Whilst for addition, you can put either number on top, for subtraction the order of the numbers is important. The number that you are subtracting from should be written at the top with the number that you are taking from it underneath.

For example, if you need to work out 585 – 143, it is the 585 that should be written at the top of the calculation. Again, start with the units column and work from right to left, this time taking away the numbers in that column.

$$
\begin{array}{r}
5 \quad 8 \quad 5 \\
- \quad 1 \quad 4 \quad 3 \\
\hline
\mathbf{4 \quad 4 \quad 2} \\
\hline
\end{array}
$$

In the example above, all of the subtractions were straightforward. This is not always the case. Sometimes you will need to take a larger number from a smaller one. For example, if you are asked to work out 91 – 64, you would line up the numbers according to place value.

$$
\begin{array}{r}
9 \quad 1 \\
- \quad 6 \quad 4 \\
\hline
\\
\hline
\end{array}
$$

The first subtraction that you would need to do is 1 – 4, which is not possible without going into negative numbers (which would not help in a problem like this).

The way around this is to 'borrow' 1 from the next column. This is taking one of your 'tens' and changing it into 10 units, which would mean that instead of having 9 tens and 1 unit, you now have 8 tens and 11 units. You can then subtract as before.

$$
\begin{array}{r}
9^{8} \quad {}^{1}1 \\
\cdot \quad 6 \quad 4 \\
\hline
\mathbf{2 \quad 7} \\
\hline
\end{array}
$$

The answer to this question is 27.

Have a Go

Work out 315 – 184

You may sometimes be in a situation where you need to borrow, but there is nothing in the next column to borrow from.

For example, you may be trying to work out 303 – 187.

$$
\begin{array}{r}
3\ \ 0\ \ 3 \\
-\ \ 1\ \ 8\ \ 7 \\
\hline
\\
\hline
\end{array}
$$

After you have lined up the numbers in this example, the first calculation to carry out is 3 - 7. This cannot be done, so you will need to borrow from the tens. However, there are zero tens in the top number.

You cannot borrow directly from the hundreds to the units. Instead, you must borrow one of the hundreds to become 10 tens, and borrow one of these tens (leaving 9 tens) and changing it to 10 units. You can then subtract as before.

$$
\begin{array}{r}
3^{2}\ \ {}^{1}0^{9}\ \ {}^{1}3 \\
-\ \ 1\ \ \ 8\ \ \ 7 \\
\hline
1\ \ \ 1\ \ \ 6 \\
\hline
\end{array}
$$

Have a Go

Work out 406 - 88

Subtracting Decimals

Again, a similar method can be applied to subtracting decimals. However, this time it is important not to have 'gaps' in columns (particularly the columns after the decimal point). You do not want to end up in a situation where you have a number to take away and nothing to take it from.

After lining up your numbers according to their place value, fill in any blank columns with zeroes before completing the subtraction.

For example, if you are working out 1.5 – 0.86, start by lining the number up in columns (using the decimal point as your guide).

$$
\begin{array}{r}
1\ .\ 5 \\
-\quad 0\ .\ 8\ 6 \\
\hline
. \\
\hline
\end{array}
$$

There is a blank space in the hundredths column of the top number. This needs to be filled with a zero, and then you can proceed with the subtraction as before.

$$
\begin{array}{r}
\overset{0}{1}\ .\ \overset{1}{5}{}^{4}\ \overset{1}{0} \\
-\quad 0\ .\ 8\ \ 6 \\
\hline
0\ .\ 6\ \ 4 \\
\hline
\end{array}
$$

Notice that in this instance, we needed to 'borrow' for both the hundredths and then the tenths. You can borrow as many times as you need for a given calculation.

Have a Go

Work out 1.35 – 0.046

Multiplication

Multiplying numbers comes down to two skills – knowing your times tables and understanding place value.

Learning your times tables (at least up to 10 × 10) by heart is very important in multiplication. For many people it can take time and practice but it is well worth the effort. A good method for learning your tables is to write any questions that you are not confident with on cards and regularly select from your cards randomly and attempt to answer the question.

On the next page is a times table grid to help you learn your tables.

X	1	2	3	4	5	6	7	8	9	10
1	1	2	3	4	5	6	7	8	9	10
2	2	4	6	8	10	12	14	16	18	20
3	3	6	9	12	15	18	21	24	27	30
4	4	8	12	16	20	24	28	32	36	40
5	5	10	15	20	25	30	35	40	45	50
6	6	12	18	24	30	36	42	48	54	60
7	7	14	21	28	35	42	49	56	63	70
8	8	16	24	32	40	48	56	64	72	80
9	9	18	27	36	45	54	63	72	81	90
10	10	20	30	40	50	60	70	80	90	100

Multiplying by Multiples of Powers of 10

In the previous chapter on place value, we looked at how you can multiply numbers by powers of 10 (for example 10, 100, 1000) by moving the digits of the number (move the digits 1 place to multiply by 10, 2 places to multiply by 100, 3 places to multiply by 1000, etc.)

For example, to work out 23 × 100, move each of the digits 2 places left (and fill the gaps with zeroes) for an answer of 2300.

When you are trying to multiply by a number that is a multiple of 10, you can break the calculation into two parts. First multiply by **how many tens you have**, then multiply the answer by 10.

For example, to multiply a number by 30, you can first multiply it by 3 and then multiply the answer by 10. So 7 × 30 = 7 × 3 × 10 = 21 × 10 = 210.

In a similar way, you can break down multiples of 100 or 1000 to make your multiplication calculations easier. 5 × 400 is the same as 5 × 4 × 100 = 20 × 100 = 2000.

Have a Go

Work out 6 × 800

The Grid Method

When you are confident multiplying numbers by multiples of powers of 10, then you can break any multiplication question into these building blocks, using a method known as the grid method.

To use the grid method, break the numbers that you are multiplying down into component parts, using the place value of each digit. For example, 183 would break down into 100, 80 and 3 and 67 would break down into 60 and 7.

Now write the component parts of one of the numbers you are multiplying as the column headers on a grid and the component parts of the other number as the row headers.

If you wanted to multiply together 183 and 67, your grid would look like this.

x	100	80	3
60			
7			

Now work out the value for each cell by multiplying together the column and row headers for that box. For example, the first cell would be 60 x 100 = 6000.

The rest of the grid would be filled out as follows.

x	100	80	3
60	6000	4800	180
7	700	560	21

To get the final answer, add together the values in each of the cells. 6000 + 4800 + 180 + 700 + 560 + 21 = 12261, so 183 × 67 = 12261.

Have a Go

Use the grid method to work out 219 × 54.

Decimal Multiplication

When you need to multiply together two decimal numbers, start by multiplying the numbers together as though they were not decimals.

For example, if you need to work out 6.4 × 0.85, you would ignore decimal points and work out 64 × 85 using the grid method as above.

x	60	4
80	4800	320
5	300	20

The answer to 64 × 85 is 4800 + 320 + 300 + 20 = 5440.

Once you have obtained this answer, you will need to adjust the place value of the numbers to find the answer to the original decimal calculation.

Your answer should have the same number of digits after the decimal points as the numbers in the question do (combined). In this case, 6.4 has one digit after the decimal point and 0.85 has two digits after the decimal point. This is a total of three digits after the point, so the last three of the digits in your answer will need to be written after a decimal point, giving 5.440 (which can just be written as 5.44).

Have a Go

Work out 3.6 × 13.2

Division

Division is about splitting numbers into parts. For example, if you were asked to divide a number by 4, that would mean you are splitting the number into four parts.

The method that you use for division will depend on what number you are trying to divide by. When you are dividing by a small number (10 or less), the best method is short division, also known as the bus-stop method.

To divide using this method, place the number that you want to divide on the inside of a bus stop, and the number that you are dividing by on the outside.

For example, if you want to work out 684 ÷ 9 then you would set up the 'bus-stop' as below.

$$9 \mid \overline{6 \quad 8 \quad 4}$$

When using this method, you try dividing the 9 into each of the digits in turn, working from left to right. Write how many times the 9 goes into the number on top of the bus-stop, and write the remainder before the next digit in the number to turn it into a 2-digit number.

In this case, 9 goes into 6 zero times with a remainder of six, so write 0 on top of the bus-stop, and 6 before the 8 to turn it into 68.

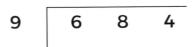

Now repeat the process for the next digit. 9 goes into 68 seven times with a remainder of five, so write 7 above the bus-stop and the 5 before the 4 to turn it into 54.

$$\begin{array}{c} 0 \qquad 7 \\ 9 \mid \overline{6 \quad {}^{6}8 \quad {}^{5}4} \end{array}$$

Finally, 9 goes into 54 exactly six times so write 6 above the bus-stop.

$$\begin{array}{c} 0 \qquad 7 \qquad 6 \\ 9 \mid \overline{6 \quad {}^{6}8 \quad {}^{5}4} \end{array}$$

This means that 684 ÷ 9 = 76.

Have a Go

Work out 592 ÷ 4

Chunking

When you are dividing by a larger number, you will probably need to use another method that is known as chunking.

In this method, you subtract 'chunks' of the number that you are dividing by. These chunks would usually be 100, 10, 5, 2 or 1 lot of the number.

For example, if you want to work out 544 ÷ 32, start by taking away the largest 'chunk' of 32 that you can. 100 × 32 would be 3200, so take away 10 × 32 (=320). At the side of the calculation, make a note of how many 32s have been taken away.

$$
\begin{array}{c|ccc}
32 & 5 & 4 & 4 & \\
- & 3 & 2 & 0 & \mathbf{10} \\
\hline
 & 2 & 2 & 4 &
\end{array}
$$

The remainder is 224. This is not enough to take away another chunk of 320, so this time take away 5 × 32 (=160).

$$
\begin{array}{c|ccc}
32 & 5 & 4 & 4 & \\
- & 3 & 2 & 0 & \mathbf{10} \\
\hline
 & 2 & 2 & 4 & \\
 & 1 & 6 & 0 & \mathbf{5} \\
\hline
 & & 6 & 4 &
\end{array}
$$

Finally, you can take away a chunk of 2 × 32 (=64), which will leave a remainder of zero.

$$
\begin{array}{r|ccc}
32 & 5 & 4 & 4 \\
\hline
- & 3 & 2 & 0 \qquad \mathbf{10} \\
\hline
& 2 & 2 & 4 \\
& 1 & 6 & 0 \qquad \mathbf{5} \\
\hline
& & 6 & 4 \\
& & 6 & 4 \qquad \mathbf{2} \\
\hline
& & & 0
\end{array}
$$

Count up how many 32s you have taken away in total and this will be the final answer. In this case, 10 + 5 + 2 = 17, so 544 ÷ 32 = 17.

Have a Go

Use the chunking method to work out 468 ÷ 18

The Fractions Method

An alternative to chunking is the fractions method.

To divide using this method, set up the two numbers in your calculation as a fraction, with the number that you are dividing on the top and the number you are dividing by on the bottom.

In the example above, the fraction you use would be $\frac{544}{32}$.

Simplify this fraction (for more on how to do this see the chapter on fractions). If you can manage to simplify the fraction so there is a one on the bottom of the fraction, then the top number of the fraction will be the answer to your calculation.

$\frac{544}{32}$ can be simplified by (repeatedly) dividing both numbers by 2.

$$^{544}/_{32} = {}^{272}/_{16} = {}^{136}/_{8} = {}^{68}/_{4} = {}^{34}/_{2} = {}^{17}/_{1}$$

The answer is 17 as before.

Have a Go

Use the fractions method to work out 468 ÷ 18.

Did you get the same answer as before?

Which method do you prefer?

Dividing with Decimals

The fractions method can be particularly helpful when one (or both) of the numbers in the question are decimals.

When this happens, you can use equivalent fractions to repeatedly multiply both numbers by 10 until the calculation only contains whole numbers and then work out the answer as before.

For example, if you need to work out 3.6 ÷ 0.24, set up the calculation as a fraction, which would be $^{3.6}/_{0.24}$.

When you multiply both numbers by 10, this leaves $^{36}/_{2.4}$. As there is still a decimal in this calculation, multiply by 10 again to get $^{360}/_{24}$ and then solve by simplifying the fraction as before.

$$^{360}/_{24} = {}^{180}/_{12} = {}^{90}/_{6} = {}^{45}/_{3} = {}^{15}/_{1}$$

The answer is 15.

Have a Go

Work out 10.8 ÷ 0.27

Whichever method you use, it is possible that the number you are dividing by will not go into the number exactly. In this case, the answer will be a decimal. You will usually have access to a calculator if you need to perform a division with a decimal answer. Using short division or chunking will give you an answer with a remainder, which is a good guide to what the scale of your answer should be (the fractions method will not do this – but when you have simplified the fraction as far as you can you could divide the numbers that remain using either short division or chunking).

Practice Questions

Question 1

What is 728 + 195?

Question 2

What is 27.2 + 1.835?

Question 3

What is 806 - 279?

Question 4

What is 48.1 – 3.65?

Question 5

What is 38 × 476?

Question 6

What is 9.3 × 28?

Question 7

What is 7.61 × 0.84?

Question 8

What is 942 ÷ 6?

Question 9

What is 1824 ÷ 48?

Question 10

What is 12.96 ÷ 1.44?

Solutions

Fully worked solutions to all of these questions can be accessed at *www.mathsfornurses.com/calculations*

Have a Go

1. 452

2. 3.835

3. 131

4. 318

5. 1.304

6. 4800

7. 11826

8. 47.52

9. 148

10. 26

11. 40

Practice Questions

1. 923

2. 29.035

3. 527

4. 44.45

5. 18088

6. 260.4

7. 6.3924

8. 157

9. 38

10. 9

Rounding Numbers

In many situations, it can be helpful to round your answer to a certain level of accuracy. For example, it is unlikely that you would describe the weight of a child as 32.41896442608kg. Instead, you would approximate the number to 32kg (or perhaps 32.4kg) to make it easier to work with.

In different contexts, you may need to round a number to the nearest thousand, to the nearest hundred, to the nearest ten, to the nearest whole number, to a given number of decimal places or to a given number of significant figures.

Rounding to the Nearest 1000, 100 or 10

If you are asked to round to the nearest ten, the nearest hundred or the nearest thousand, you need to identify the digit in question and place a partition after that digit.

For example, if you are asked to round 2475 to the nearest hundred, the hundreds digit is '4', so place the partition after this digit.

$$2 \quad 4 \mid 7 \quad 5$$

Look at the digit immediately to the right of the partition.

If the digit is less than five, leave what is to the left of the partition as it is and replace everything to the right of the partition with zeroes.

If the digit is five or more, increase what is to the left of the partition by 1 and replace what is to the right of the partition with zeroes.

In the example above, the digit to the right of the partition is '7', and so because this is greater than five, the number to the left of the partition increases by 1, from 24 to 25 and to the right of the partition, the 75 becomes 00, giving an answer of 2500.

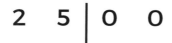

$$2 \quad 5 \mid 0 \quad 0$$

Have a Go

Round 2475 (a) to the nearest thousand, and (b) to the nearest ten.

Rounding to the Nearest Whole Number

When you want to round a number to the nearest whole number, you need to put the partition where the decimal point is. The process will be the same as above, but instead of putting zeroes to the right of the partition, just delete everything to the right of it.

For example, round 6.25 to the nearest whole number.

$$6 \mid 2 \; 5$$

The partition would be on the decimal point, so the next digit is a '2'. Because this is less than 5, keep everything left of the partition as it is (6 in this case) and get rid of everything right of the partition (the 2 and the 5), so the final answer would just be 6.

If you wanted to round 3.74 to the nearest whole number, the digit after the partition would be a '7'.

$$3 \mid 7 \; 4$$

In this case, the digit is greater than a 5 so increase the number to the left of the partition by 1 from 3 to 4 and get rid of everything to the right of the partition (the 7 and the 4), so the final answer will be 4.

Have a Go

Round 7.06 to the nearest whole number.

Rounding to Decimal Places

Sometimes you will be asked to round a number to 1 decimal place or 2 decimal places (or more).

In this situation, put the partition the specified number of places after the decimal point, and then follow the same process for rounding to the nearest whole number.

For example, if you are asked to round 6.25 to 1 decimal place, the partition would need to go one place after the decimal point (as shown below).

$$6 \ . \ 2 \ | \ 5$$

The digit after the partition is a 5, and because 5 rounds up, increase the number to the left of the partition from 6.2 to 6.3. Everything to the right of the partition disappears, so the final answer is 6.3.

Similarly, to round 1.074 to two decimal places, the partition would need to go two places after the decimal point, which would leave it between the '7' and the '4' as shown below.

$$1 \ . \ 0 \ 7 \ | \ 4$$

The digit to the right of the partition is less than a 5, so you can leave the number to the left of the partition as it is and get rid of everything to the right of the partition to leave an answer of 1.07.

Have a Go

Round 8.463 to (a) 1 decimal place and (b) 2 decimal places.

It is possible that when you round a number to a given number of decimal places up, the digit that you will need to increase is a '9'. For example, if you need to round 1.96 to 1 decimal place you would place your partition between the 9 and the 6 as shown below.

$$1 \ . \ 9 \ | \ 6$$

Because the '6' is larger than 5 you will need to round up, but you cannot increase the 9 to 10 and make the answer '1.10'. Instead, consider the 1.9 as a whole and round it up to 2.0. Then discard everything to the right of the partition, so the final answer will be 2.0.

Rounding to Significant Figures

As well as rounding to decimal places, it is also possible to round to significant figures.

This works in a similar way to rounding to a given number of decimal places, but instead of counting digits from the decimal point, you count from the first digit of the number that is not a zero.

For example, round 7.486 to 2 significant figures. The first digit of the number is the 7, so place the partition 2 places from this digit, as shown below.

$$7 \ . \ 4 \ | \ 8 \ 6$$

Once you have placed the partition you can round as before. The digit to the right of the partition is greater than a 5, so you would increase the number to the left of the partition to 7.5 and discard everything to the right of the partition.

As another example, round 0.000365 to 1 significant figure.

The partition needs to be placed after the first digit that is not a zero (in this case the '3') as shown below.

$$0 \ . \ 0 \ 0 \ 0 \ 3 \ | \ 6 \ 5$$

The digit to the left of the partition is greater than 5 so increase the number to the left of the partition from 0.0003 to 0.0004 and discard everything to the right of the partition for a final answer of 0.0004.

In the context of drug calculations, it is usual to round answers to 2 decimal places, though in different contexts there will be different degrees of accuracy required and it is important to be familiar with all the different ways of rounding numbers.

Practice Questions on Rounding

Question 1

Round 7146 to the nearest hundred.

Question 2

Round 1895 to the nearest ten.

Question 3

Round 11.64 to the nearest whole number.

Question 4

Round 24.68 to the nearest ten.

Question 5

Round 7.37 to one decimal place.

Question 6

Round 0.082175 to two decimal places.

Question 7

Round 8.995 to two decimal places.

Question 8

Round 42.1396 to three significant figures.

Question 9

Round 2.491 to two significant figures.

Question 10

Round 0.002867 to three significant figures.

Solutions

Fully worked solutions to all of these questions can be accessed at www.mathsfornurses.com/roundingnumbers

Have a Go

1. a) 2000 & b) 2480

2. 7

3. a) 8.5 & b) 8.46

Practice Questions

1. 7100

2. 1900

3. 12

4. 20

5. 7.4

6. 0.08

7. 9.00

8. 42.1

9. 2.5

10. 0.00287

Converting Measurements

One of the most frequently used numeracy skills in nursing is the ability to convert measurements from one unit to another. For example, a patient may be prescribed a drug in milligrams and the amount of the drug in each tablet is measured in micrograms. You need to know how to convert between these two units of measure.

The Metric System

Since the 1970s, the UK has used the metric system of measures. This system is designed to make conversions easier because you will be multiplying and dividing by 10, 100 and 1000 (rather than 12, 14 and 16 as in the old system).

In the metric system, there is a base unit for each type of measurement, that is then scaled up or down by attaching a prefix to that unit.

Common base units include 'metre' for length, 'gram' for weight and 'litre' for capacity.

There are prefixes for these base units that can scale them up or down by any power of ten. For our purposes, we only need to focus on those prefixes that scale a number up or down by 1000.

- **KILO** – means that the unit is multiplied by 1000. For example, a kilometre is a thousand metres and a kilogram is a thousand grams.

- **MILLI** – means that the unit is divided by 1000. For example, a thousand milligrams make a gram and a thousand millilitres make a litre.

- **MICRO** – means that the unit is divided by 1000 again. For example, a thousand micrograms make a milligram (which would mean that it takes a million micrograms to make a gram).

- **NANO** – means that the unit is divided by 1000 one more time. For example, a thousand nanograms make a microgram (which would mean that it takes a billion nanograms to make a gram).

Weights & Capacities

In the nursing context, the measurements that you are most likely to use are weights and capacities.

The main measures of weight that you need to be familiar with are kilograms (kg), grams (g), milligrams (mg), micrograms (µg – or sometimes referred to as mcg) and nanograms (ng). The conversions between these units are shown in the diagram below.

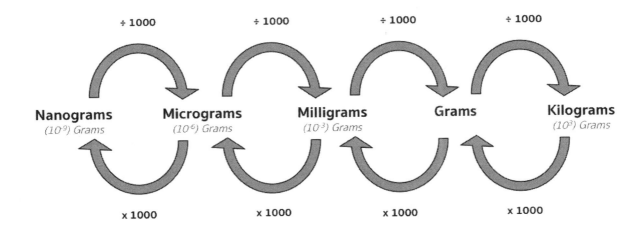

When working with units of capacity, you will probably only need to use litres (L or l) and millilitres (mL or ml). The conversions between these units are shown below.

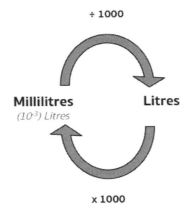

Converting From a Larger Unit to a Smaller One

When you need to convert a measurement from a larger unit to a smaller one, the method you use is to multiply the number by the conversion factor (in the examples that we are considering, this will be 1000).

For example, the conversion factor for converting from litres to millilitres is 1000, so to convert 2.8 litres into millilitres you will need to multiply 2.8 by 1000 (an explanation of how to do this can be found in the 'Place Value' chapter) to get an answer of 2800ml.

Similarly, the conversion factor for converting micrograms into nanograms is also 1000. If you need to convert 0.8 micrograms into nanograms, work out 0.8 × 1000 = 800 nanograms.

Have a Go

Convert 4.5 milligrams into micrograms.

Converting From a Smaller Unit to a Larger One

When you need to convert a measurement from a smaller unit to a larger one, rather than multiply by the conversion factor you need to divide by it.

For example, the conversion factor for converting grams into kilograms is 1000. If you need to convert 4000 grams into kilograms, work out 4000 ÷ 1000 = 4 kg (again, there is an explanation of how to divide by 1000 in the 'Place Value' chapter).

Similarly, to convert 700 micrograms into milligrams, work out 700 ÷ 1000 = 0.7 milligrams.

Have a Go

Convert 1250 millilitres into litres.

Two-Step Conversions

Occasionally you may need to convert a measurement from one unit to a unit that is considerably larger or smaller.

For example, you may wish to convert 8500 micrograms into grams.

As it is much more common to convert measurements from micrograms into milligrams and to convert from milligrams into grams, the easiest way to convert from micrograms into grams would be to go through the intermediate step of first converting into milligrams.

Convert 8500 micrograms into milligrams by dividing it by 1000. This gives 8.5mg. Then divide this answer by 1000 again to convert it into grams. 8.5 ÷ 1000 = 0.0085, so 8500µg is the same as 0.0085g.

Have a Go

Convert 0.07kg into milligrams.

Practice Questions on Converting Measurements

Question 1

Convert 5 litres into millilitres.

Question 2

Convert 12 milligrams into micrograms.

Question 3

Convert 14.2 kilograms into grams.

Question 4

Convert 0.34 grams into milligrams.

Question 5

Convert 2000 grams into kilograms.

Question 6

Convert 1200mL into litres.

Question 7

Convert 800µg into milligrams.

Question 8

Convert 420ng into micrograms.

Question 9

Convert 15000mg into kilograms.

Question 10

Convert 0.002g into micrograms.

Solutions

Fully worked solutions to all of these questions can be accessed at www.mathsfornurses.com/convertingmeasurements

Have a Go

1. 4500µg

2. 1.25L

3. 70000mg

Practice Questions

1. 5000mL

2. 12000µg

3. 14200g

4. 340mg

5. 2kg

6. 1.2L

7. 0.8mg

8. 0.42µg

9. 0.015kg

10. 2000µg

Fractions

Fractions, decimals, and percentages are three different ways of expressing the same thing. Each of them can tell you how many parts you have of a whole. This is called proportion. It is important that you know how to work with each in its own right, and that you are able to convert between them.

A fraction is made up of 2 numbers. The top number (known as the numerator) tells you how many parts you have, and the bottom number (the denominator) tells you how many parts there are altogether.

For example, the fraction $^2/_7$ means that out of 7 parts altogether, you have 2. A possible context for such a fraction arising would be if out of 7 beds on a ward, 2 were available. Because there are 2 parts out of a total of 7, the fraction of beds that is available is $^2/_7$.

The Simplest Form of a Fraction

Sometimes you will be asked to give a fraction in its 'simplest form' or 'lowest terms'. Different fractions can mean the same thing, and you want to give the fraction that uses the lowest numbers to express it. For example, saying that two patients out of twelve have a reaction to a particular medicine is the same as saying that one patient out of every six has the reaction. The fractions $^2/_{12}$ and $^1/_6$ mean the same thing, but $^1/_6$ expresses it using smaller numbers, so this is the fraction in its lowest terms.

To work out a fraction in its lowest terms, you need to see if there is a number that you could divide both the numerator and the denominator by, and still get whole numbers as the answers. If there is, divide by that number. This is simplifying the fraction. Then check whether you can simplify your new fraction again. When the fraction cannot be simplified any more, it is in its simplest form. For example, you may need to write the fraction $^{24}/_{36}$ in its simplest form. You notice that both numbers can be divided by 4, and this would leave you with $^6/_9$. Now you notice that both of the numbers in your new fraction can be divided by 3, giving an answer of $^2/_3$. This cannot be simplified any more so $^2/_3$ is the fraction in its lowest terms.

Have a Go

What is the simplest form of $^{30}/_{42}$?

Finding a Fraction of Amount

Often you will be given a fraction and asked to work out that proportion of a given quantity.

To calculate this, your first step is to divide the number by the denominator of the fraction (this is splitting the whole up into parts), and your second step is to multiply your answer to the first step by the numerator of the fraction (choosing how many parts you want).

For example, if 30 medical students are invited to an optional seminar and $^2/_5$ of those students turned up, you may need to calculate how many students are present.

Start by dividing 30 by the denominator. $30 \div 5 = 6$. Multiply this answer by the numerator of the fraction. $6 \times 2 = 12$. 12 students are present at the seminar.

Have a Go

A child's dose of a medicine is $^3/_8$ of the adult dose. If the adult dose is 120mg, what is the child's dose?

If you are asked to find a fraction of an amount, you will find the calculations much easier if you put the fraction into its lowest terms first. For example, if you need to find $^{12}/_{15}$ of a number, instead of dividing by 15 and multiplying the answer by 12, you could simplify your fraction to $^4/_5$, then you only have to divide by 5 and multiply by 4, which will give you easier calculations to work out.

Adding & Subtracting Fractions

It is possible to add or subtract two fractions together. In order to do this, both fractions must have the whole divided into pieces of the same size. This means that the denominators of both fractions need to be the same. For example, you could add $^3/_5$ and $^1/_5$ together but you could not add $^3/_5$ and $^1/_4$.

When you are adding two fractions with the same denominator, the answer will have the same denominator too and you simply add together the two numerators in the question. For example $^3/_5 + ^1/_5 = ^{(3+1)}/_5 = ^4/_5$.

In a similar way, when you are subtracting fractions you leave the denominator the same and subtract the two numerators. $^3/_5 - ^1/_5 = ^{(3-1)}/_5 = ^2/_5$.

Have a Go

Work out $2/7 + 4/7$

Have a Go

Work out $7/8 - 3/8$

If you do need to add or subtract fractions with different denominators, you need to first convert both of the fractions to equivalent fractions with the same denominator as each other.

Consider the example of $3/5 + 1/4$. You will need to choose a denominator for your new fractions that both of the existing denominators divide into. The lowest number that is in both the fives times table and the four times table is 20, so you need to find equivalent fractions with 20 as the denominator.

To find an equivalent fraction, multiply the numerator and denominator by the same thing. $3/5$ needs to have both terms multiplied by 4 to end up with a denominator of 20, This would give the fraction $12/20$.

$1/4$ would need to have both terms multiplied by 5 to end up with a denominator of 20, which would give the fraction $5/20$.

You can now add these new fractions together as before. $12/20 + 5/20 = 17/20$.

Have a Go

Work out $1/2 + 2/5$

Have a Go

Work out $5/6 - 3/4$

Multiplying Fractions

If you need to multiply two fractions together, you can do this by multiplying the numerators together and multiplying the denominators together. You may then need to simplify your answer.

For example, if you want to work out $\frac{1}{4} \times \frac{2}{3}$, you need to work out $1 \times 2 = 2$ for the numerator and $4 \times 3 = 12$ for the denominator, meaning that the answer will be $\frac{2}{12}$, which can then be simplified to $\frac{1}{6}$.

Have a Go

Work out $\frac{1}{6} \times \frac{3}{4}$

Dividing Fractions

Dividing fractions follows a similar method to multiplying fractions but you first need to 'flip' the second fraction in the calculation upside down (i.e. swap the numerator and the denominator around). Once you have done this, you can **multiply** as before.

For example, if you want to work out $\frac{1}{4} \div \frac{2}{3}$, start by flipping the second fraction and replacing the division symbol with a multiplication one. This means that your calculation will become $\frac{1}{4} \times \frac{3}{2}$, which you can work out as before to get an answer of $\frac{3}{8}$.

Have a Go

Work out $\frac{1}{6} \div \frac{3}{4}$

Practice Questions on Fractions

Question 1

Write $\frac{9}{12}$ in its simplest form.

Question 2

Write $\frac{14}{42}$ in its simplest form.

Question 3

What is $\frac{5}{8}$ of 48?

Question 4

An infant needs to take $5/12$ of an adult dose of a medicine. If the adult dose is 60ml, how much should the infant take?

Question 5

Work out $5/9 + 2/9$.

Question 6

Work out $2/3 - 1/4$.

Question 7

Work out $1/7 \times 3/4$.

Question 8

Work out $9/10 \times 2/3$. Give your answer in its simplest form.

Question 9

Work out $2/3 \div 3/4$.

Question 10

Work out $1/5 \div 4/5$. Give your answer in its simplest form.

Solutions

Fully worked solutions to all of these questions can be accessed at <u>*www.mathsfornurses.com/fractions*</u>

Have a Go

1. $^5/_7$

2. 45mg

3. $^6/_7$

4. $^4/_8$

5. $^9/_{10}$

6. $^1/_{12}$

7. $^3/_{24}$

8. $^2/_9$

Practice Questions

1. $^3/_4$

2. $^1/_3$

3. 30

4. 25ml

5. $^7/_9$

6. $^5/_{12}$

7. $^3/_{28}$

8. $^3/_5$

9. $^8/_9$

10. $^1/_4$

Converting Fractions, Decimals & Percentages

You sometimes need to express proportions in different forms. To do this, you will need to be able to convert between fractions, decimals and percentages.

Some conversions are very common, and you may find it helpful to memorise them. These are shown on the table below.

Fraction	$\frac{1}{100}$	$\frac{1}{20}$	$\frac{1}{10}$	$\frac{1}{8}$	$\frac{1}{5}$	$\frac{1}{4}$	$\frac{1}{3}$	$\frac{2}{5}$	$\frac{1}{2}$	$\frac{3}{5}$	$\frac{2}{3}$	$\frac{3}{4}$	$\frac{4}{5}$
Decimal	0.01	0.05	0.1	0.125	0.2	0.25	0.33...	0.4	0.5	0.6	0.66...	0.75	0.8
Percentage	1%	5%	10%	12.5%	20%	25%	33.3%	40%	50%	60%	66.7%	75%	80%

If you are asked a multiple of one of these, you can use the conversion you know multiplied by your new numerator. For example, if you need to work out $^3/_8$ as a percentage and you have memorised that $^1/_8 = 12.5\%$, then you can do $12.5 \times 3 = 37.5\%$.

Have a Go

What is $^3/_{20}$ as a decimal?

Other times, you will need to convert fractions, decimals or percentages that are not included in the table. A good starting point in this is to understand how these different ways of expressing proportion work.

When you have a fraction, the bottom number tells you how many the 'whole' is and the top number tells you how many parts you have. With a percentage, you take the whole to be 100 and the percentage you have is the number of parts out of that 100. If you are working with a decimal, you are expressing what part you have out of a whole of '1'.

Starting With a Percentage

When you start with a percentage, you are told how many parts you have out of 100. For example, 62% means 62 parts out of every 100.

If you want to convert a percentage to a fraction, you need to put 100 as the denominator and the percentage you have been given as the numerator. In our example, 62% can be written as $^{62}/_{100}$ and can then be simplified to its lowest terms, giving $^{31}/_{50}$.

To convert a percentage to a decimal, you will need to divide it by 100. You do this by moving each digit two places to the right, so 62% will become 0.62.

Have a Go

Write 45% as a fraction (in simplest terms) and as a decimal.

Starting With a Decimal

If you are given a decimal, you are expressing how many parts you have out of each whole '1'. To change this to a percentage you will need to find parts per hundred, so multiply your decimal by 100. This is the opposite of dividing by 100, so you will need to move each digit two places left. For example, 0.89 will be 89%.

To convert the decimal to a fraction, you will first need to decide your denominator. Count how many digits are after the decimal point. If there is one digit, use 10 as the denominator. If there are two digits, use 100 and if there are 3 digits use 1000. For each extra digit, you will need to add an extra zero to your denominator. Use the digits after the decimal point as your numerator. If, for example, your decimal is 0.55, you have two digits after the decimal point so the denominator is 100 and the numerator will be 55. This gives you $^{55}/_{100}$, which can be simplified to $^{11}/_{20}$.

Have a Go

Write 0.32 as a percentage and as a fraction (in simplest terms).

Particular care should be taken with decimals that are just one digit after the decimal place (such as 0.6), as this will become 60% when written as a percentage (a common mistake would be to write 6%). Also, watch out for decimals with extra zeroes after the decimal point such as 0.05. When written as a fraction this will be $^{5}/_{100}$, not $^{5}/_{10}$ and can be simplified to $^{1}/_{20}$.

Have a Go

Write 0.3 as a percentage and as a fraction (in simplest terms).

Have a Go

Write 0.02 as a percentage and as a fraction (in simplest terms).

Starting With a Fraction

When you start with a fraction, you can convert it to a percentage by finding an equivalent fraction that has 100 as the denominator. To do this, you need to multiply both numbers in the fraction by the same thing, to end up with something out of 100. The numerator of your new fraction will be your percentage.

For example, if you need to convert $^{13}/_{25}$ into a percentage, you can multiply both numbers by 4 (you do this because multiplying 25 by 4 will give you a denominator of 100).

$^{13}/_{25} \times {}^{4}/_{4} = {}^{52}/_{100}$, so it is 52%.

If you want to convert the fraction to a decimal, first find an equivalent fraction with a denominator of 10, 100 or 1000. If your denominator is 10, use the numerator in the first place after your decimal point. If the denominator is 100, place the numerator so that it ends in the second place after your decimal point. If the denominator is 1000, place the numerator so that it ends in the third place after your decimal point.

For example, if you need to convert $^{3}/_{5}$ to a decimal, you can find an equivalent fraction with 10 on the bottom if you multiply both numbers by 2. This gives $^{6}/_{10}$. As the denominator is 10, you put the 6 in the place immediately after the decimal point, giving 0.6.

Have a Go

Express $^{7}/_{20}$ as a decimal and as a percentage.

Sometimes you may need to convert a fraction to a percentage or a decimal where the denominator will not go into 100. For example, you may have to turn $^{72}/_{80}$ into a percentage. If you need to convert a fraction like this, you should start by putting the fraction in its lowest terms and then seeing if you can turn the denominator to 100. Both numbers in $^{72}/_{80}$ can be divided by 8, giving $^{9}/_{10}$. Then multiply both numbers by 10 to give $^{90}/_{100}$, which as a percentage is 90%.

Have a Go

Express $^{51}/_{60}$ as a decimal and as a percentage.

There are times where this will not help. You will need to change a fraction to a decimal or percentage and even if you simplify the fraction, you will not be able to make the denominator into 10, 100 or 1000. For example, you may need to express $^{2}/_{7}$ as a decimal. To do so, use a calculator to divide the numerator by the denominator. $2 \div 7 = 0.29$ (rounded to 2 decimal places). If you wanted to convert this into a percentage, the process is the same but you will then need to multiply the result by 100, giving 29%.

Have a Go

Express $^{4}/_{11}$ as a decimal (to 2 decimal places) and as a percentage (to the nearest whole number).

Practice Questions on Converting Fractions, Decimals & Percentages

Question 1

Convert $^{7}/_{8}$ to a percentage.

Question 2

Convert 28% to a fraction in its simplest form.

Question 3

Convert 9% to a decimal.

Question 4

Convert 0.65 to a fraction in its simplest form.

Question 5

Convert 0.1 to a percentage.

Question 6

Convert $^2/_5$ to a decimal.

Question 7

Convert $^3/_4$ to a percentage.

Question 8

Convert $^{21}/_{70}$ to a decimal.

Question 9

Convert $^5/_6$ to a decimal (to 2 decimal places)

Question 10

Convert $^9/_{13}$ to a percentage (to the nearest whole number)

Solutions

Fully worked solutions to all of these questions can be accessed at *www.mathsfornurses.com/convertingfdp*

Have a Go

1. 0.15

2. $^9/_{20}$ & 0.45

3. 32% & $^8/_{25}$

4. 30% & $^3/_{10}$

5. 2% & $^1/_{50}$

6. 0.35 & 35%

7. 0.85 & 85%

8. 0.36 & 36%

Practice Questions

1. 87.5%

2. $^7/_{25}$

3. 0.09

4. $^{13}/_{20}$

5. 10%

6. 0.4

7. 75%

8. 0.3

9. 0.83

10. 69%

Percentages

Percentages are a way of expressing a proportion as a number of parts per hundred. For example, if a solution is 50% dextrose it means that out of every 100 parts, 50 of them (i.e. half of them) are dextrose. If a different solution is 5% dextrose, then only 5 parts out of every 100 are dextrose, so it is a much more dilute solution.

Often you will need to work out a particular percentage of an amount. There are certain percentages that are easy to find, and you can use these easy percentages as building blocks to find any other percentage that you require.

*   **50%** - This is another way of saying half, so to find 50% of a number, you can divide it by 2.

*   **25%** - This is another way of saying a quarter, so to find 25% of a number, you can divide it by 4.

*   **10%** - This is one tenth of a number, so to find 10% of a number you can divide it by 10.

*   **1%** - This is one hundredth of a number, so to find 1% of a number you can divide it by 100.

For example, to find 50% of 680, you can work out 680 ÷ 2 = 340, to find 25% of 680 work out 680 ÷ 4 = 170, to find 10% of 680 work out 680 ÷ 10 = 68 and to find 1% of 680 work out 680 ÷ 100 = 6.8.

Have a Go

Work out: (a) 50% of 140; (b) 25% of 140; (c) 10% of 140; (d) 1% of 140.

Using these basic percentages as building blocks, you can work out any other percentage.

For example, you could work out 62% of 680 by recognising that 62% is the same as 50% + 10% + 1% + 1%. We have already worked out these building blocks, so we can find that 62% of 680 = 340 + 68 + 6.8 + 6.8 = 421.6.

Have a Go

Work out 87% of 140.

Alternative Method

If you have access to a calculator, an alternative way of working out a percentage is to divide the number that you start with by 100, and multiply the answer by the percentage that you are trying to find.

In the example above, this would mean using your calculator to work out $680 \div 100 \times 62$ and would give the same answer as before, 421.6.

Have a Go

Try using this alternative method to work out 87% of 140.

Did you get the same answer as before?

Which method do you prefer? (It is important to be comfortable with both methods as you may not always have a calculator available).

Percentage Increase & Decrease

In some situations, you will need to increase or decrease an amount by a given percentage.

In both of these cases, you would start by calculating the required percentage (as above). If you are working out a percentage increase you would then add this answer on to the amount you started with. To work out a percentage decrease, you would take it away from your starting amount.

For example, if you want to increase 320 by 35%, start by working out 35% of 320. 25% is 80, and 10% is 32, so 35% is 112. The final answer for the percentage increase will be 320 + 112 = 432.

As another example, decrease 1500 by 17%. Start by working out 17% of 1500.

$1500 \div 100 \times 17 = 255$.

Because we are working out a percentage decrease, the final calculation will be 1500 – 255 = 1245.

Have a Go

Increase 75 by 20%.

Have a Go

Decrease 360 by 57%.

Writing One Number as a Percentage of Another

You may need to work out what percentage one number is of another. For example, if a patient is prescribed 60ml of a medicine and has already been administered 15ml, you may want to work out what percentage has been administered already.

To do this, divide the amount that you are trying to work out by the total amount (this will give the proportion as a decimal) and then multiply the answer by 100 to turn it into a percentage.

In this example, the percentage already administered would be 15 ÷ 60 × 100 = 25%.

Have a Go

A baby is born weighing 2.1kg. What percentage is this of the average birth weight of 3.5kg?

Practice Questions on Percentages

Question 1

Without using a calculator, find 10% of 82.

Question 2

Without using a calculator, find 24% of 310.

Question 3

Find 17% of 954.

Question 4

Find 91% of 134.62

Question 5

Increase 180 by 25%.

Question 6

Increase 715 by 26%.

Question 7

Decrease 115 by 20%.

Question 8

Decrease 219 by 33%.

Question 9

What is 18 as a percentage of 45?

Question 10

What is 72 as a percentage of 6000?

Solutions

Fully worked solutions to all of these questions can be accessed at *www.mathsfornurses.com/percentages*

Have a Go

1. (a) 70; (b) 35; (c) 14; (d) 1.4

2. 121.8

3. 90

4. 154.8

5. 60%

Practice Questions

1. 8.2

2. 74.4

3. 162.18

4. 122.5042

5. 225

6. 900.9

7. 92

8. 146.73

9. 40%

10. 1.2%

Ratio

Whereas proportions (such as fractions, decimals, and percentages) are ways of comparing one part of something to the whole, ratios compare one part directly with another part and are written with the numbers separated by a colon.

For example, if there are 3 male patients and 9 female patients in a GP's waiting room, you could say that the fraction of male patients is $^3/_{12}$ (i.e. the number of male patients out of the total number of patients), or you could express the number of male patients to the number of female patients as the ratio 3:9 (i.e. comparing the two parts directly).

It is possible to simplify a ratio just as you can simplify a fraction. In the example above, the ratio 3:9 means that for every 3 male patients there are 9 female patients. Another way of saying this is that for every male patient there are 3 female patients, so the ratio 3:9 can be simplified to 1:3.

In order to work this out, find a number that you can divide both numbers in the ratio by, and what you have left when you have divided them will be the simplified ratio. Continue to do this until you can't simplify it any more and still get whole numbers as the answers.

For example, to simplify 45:75, you could start by dividing both of the numbers by 5. This would leave 9:15. This can be simplified again by dividing the numbers 3 so give 3:5. As this cannot be simplified any further, the simplest form of the ratio is 3:5.

Have a Go

Simplify the ratio 24:42.

Scaling Up a Ratio

Sometimes you are given a ratio, and one of the quantities and need to work out the other one.

For example, if you wanted to dilute 100ml of a drug solution with water in the ratio 2:5, you would need to work out how much water to use.

In order to do this, work out the factor that you are scaling up the ratio by. Because, in the ratio, the drug solution is represented by the '2', and in practice you want to use 100ml, you are scaling up by 100 ÷ 2 = 50.

Now you can work out the amount of water you need by multiplying the number in the ratio that represents the water (the '5') by 50. This gives an answer of 5 × 50 = 250ml.

Note – you can know that it is the '2' that represents the drug solution and the '5' that represents the water because the numbers in a ratio correspond to things in the order they are listed in the description – the drug solution is mentioned before the water so it is represented by the first number of the ratio.

Have a Go

In a clinical trial, patients are split between those who will take a drug and those who will take the placebo in the ratio 3:2. In total, 90 patients will take the drug. How many will take the placebo?

Splitting a Number in a Ratio

There are times when you know the ratio and the total amount, but you do not know what either of the quantities will be.

For example, you may need to mix 100ml of a fluid that is made up of 2 different fluids in the ratio 1:4.

To do this, you need to work out how many 'parts' you are splitting the ratio into. There is 1 part of the first fluid, and there are 4 parts of the second fluid, making a total of 5 parts.

You can calculate the values of each of these parts by dividing the total that you need of the fluid by the number of parts. In this case, this would be 100ml ÷ 5 = 20ml.

The first fluid has just one of these parts, so will simply be 20ml. The second fluid has 4 parts so will be 20ml × 4 = 80ml.

You can check your answer by adding these two values together, and they should make the total that you were given in the question. 20ml + 80ml = 100ml, so we can be confident that this answer is correct.

Have a Go

Split 240 in the ratio 5:3.

Practice Questions on Ratio

Question 1

Simplify the ratio 8:6.

Question 2

Simplify the ratio 12:20

Question 3

Simplify the ratio 36:72

Question 4

In a ward, occupied beds to empty beds are in the ratio 5:1. There are 7 empty beds. How many beds are occupied?

Question 5

150ml of drug solution is mixed with water in the ratio 3:7. How much water is used?

Question 6

Scale 15mg of a drug up in the ratio 3:20.

Question 7

900ml of glucose solution is mixed with water in the ratio 6:1. How much water is used?

Question 8

Split 56 in the ratio 3:4

Question 9

Split 200ml in the ratio 3:7

Question 10

Split 450g in the ratio 11:4

Solutions

Fully worked solutions to all of these questions can be accessed at www.mathsfornurses.com/ratio

Have a Go

1. 4:7

2. 60

3. 150 & 90

Practice Questions

1. 4:3

2. 3:5

3. 1:2

4. 35

5. 350ml

6. 100mg

7. 150ml

8. 24 and 32

9. 60ml and 140ml

10. 330g and 120g

Practice Test A

Question 1

Scale 20mg up in the ratio 1:4.

Question 2

Convert $^2/_5$ to a decimal.

Question 3

Decrease 900 by 20%

Question 4

What is $^{42}/_{63}$ in its simplest form?

Question 5

Convert 6200ml into litres.

Question 6

What is 0.17 × 1000?

Question 7

What is 25.92 ÷ 1.44?

Question 8

Round 126.42 to the nearest ten.

Question 9

What percentage of 80 is 24?

Question 10

What is 84% as a fraction in its simplest form?

Question 11

Put these numbers in order from smallest to largest: 1.2, 0.62, 1.26, 1.06

Question 12

Simplify the ratio 15:35

Solutions

Worked solutions to test A can be accessed at www.mathsfornurses.com/practicetestsa-d

1. 80mg

2. 0.4

3. 720

4. $\frac{2}{3}$

5. 6.2L

6. 170

7. 18

8. 130

9. 30%

10. $\frac{21}{25}$

11. 0.62, 1.06, 1.2, 1.26

12. 3:7

Practice Test B

Question 1

What is the value of the 3 in 7231.68?

Question 2

Round 1.467 to 2 decimal places.

Question 3

What is $^2/_5$ of 45?

Question 4

What is 70% of 150?

Question 5

What is 467.12 × 10?

Question 6

Split 160 in the ratio 6:4.

Question 7

What is 1863 + 757?

Question 8

Convert 4000µg into milligrams.

Question 9

Scale 50ml up in the ratio 2:3.

Question 10

What is 0.125 as a fraction in its simplest form?

Question 11

What is 1.4 × 2.36?

Question 12

Round 749.62 to the nearest hundred.

Solutions

Worked solutions to test B can be accessed at www.mathsfornurses.com/practicetestsa-d

1. 30

2. 1.47

3. 18

4. 105

5. 4671.2

6. 96 and 64

7. 2620

8. 4mg

9. 75ml

10. $\frac{1}{8}$

11. 3.304

12. 700

Practice Test C

Question 1

What is 58 × 93?

Question 2

What percentage of 2500 is 350?

Question 3

Convert 1.3mg into µg.

Question 4

What is 3.5 ÷ 100?

Question 5

What is 0.9 as a percentage?

Question 6

Round 346.139 to 2 significant figures.

Question 7

What is 34% of 8600?

Question 8

Convert 1.75L into millilitres.

Question 9

What is $\frac{1}{7} \times \frac{5}{6}$?

Question 10

Round 2.996 to 2 decimal places.

Question 11

Simplify the ratio 4800:720.

Question 12

What is $\frac{2}{3} + \frac{1}{4}$?

Solutions

Worked solutions to test C can be accessed at www.mathsfornurses.com/practicetestsa-d

1. 5394

2. 14%

3. 1300µg

4. 0.035

5. 90%

6. 350

7. 2924

8. 1750ml

9. $\frac{5}{42}$

10. 3.00

11. 20:3

12. $\frac{11}{12}$

Practice Test D

Question 1

What is $^3/_4 - ^1/_5$?

Question 2

What is $2072 \div 28$?

Question 3

Which is larger, 8.27 or 8.3?

Question 4

Split 840g in the ratio 2:5.

Question 5

What is $^3/_4$ as a percentage?

Question 6

Increase 240 by 65%.

Question 7

What is $4102 - 1856$?

Question 8

Convert 17000µg into grams.

Question 9

Round 34.5 to the nearest whole number.

Question 10

What is $^2/_3 \div {}^1/_6$?

Question 11

What is 5% as a decimal?

Question 12

Convert 1.4g into milligrams.

Solutions

Worked solutions to test D can be accessed at www.mathsfornurses.com/practicetestsa-d

1. $^{11}/_{20}$

2. 74

3. 8.3

4. 240g and 600g

5. 75%

6. 396

7. 2246

8. 0.017g

9. 35

10. 4

11. 0.05

12. 1400mg

Calculating Dosages

Now that you have an understanding of some of the basic numeracy skills, your next step is to put these skills to use in the calculations that you will need to carry out in the context of nursing.

Drug calculations are an important part of the role of a nurse, and though these calculations can initially seem intimidating, they are actually further examples of the same numeracy skills that you have worked with in previous chapters.

To work out a required dosage, you will need to know the amount of the drug that is prescribed, and you will also need to know what amount of the drug is available in a particular 'unit' (known as the 'stock dose').

For example, a patient may have been prescribed 150 milligrams of a particular drug. The stock dose of the drug is 30mg/2ml.

This means that for every 2ml that you give to the patient, they will receive 30mg of the drug. You need to work out how much to give the patient in order for them to have 150mg of the drug.

Because the amount you need (150mg) is the same as five lots of 30mg, you will need to give the stock dose of 2ml five times, meaning the total dosage is 5 × 2 = 10ml.

In general, the method for working out these drug calculations is to divide the prescribed dose by the stock dose and multiply the answer by the volume that the stock dose is in.

Amount of Drug = Prescribed Dose ÷ Stock Dose x Volume of Stock Dose

---

Applying this method to the example above would give the calculation 150 ÷ 30 x 2 = 10ml (as before).

For another example, a patient has been prescribed 280 milligrams of a drug. The stock dose is 20mg/5ml.

To work out the dosage required, apply the numbers given into the formula above. The prescribed dose is 280mg, the stock dose is 20mg and the volume of the stock dose is 5ml.

This means that the dosage will be 280 ÷ 20 x 5 = 70ml.

Have a Go

60mg of a drug is prescribed. The stock dose is 15mg/3ml. What volume of the drug would you give?

Unit Conversions

Sometimes the prescribed dose and the stock dose may not be given in the same unit. When this is the situation, you need to convert them both into the same unit (it is better to convert them into the smaller unit so that you will end up working with whole numbers rather than with decimals).

For example, if the prescribed dose of a drug is 2mg, and the stock dose is 500µg/ml, you would need to start by converting the 2mg into 2000µg. You can then work out the required dosage as before. 2000 ÷ 500 × 1 = 4ml.

Have a Go

1.5mg of a drug is prescribed. The stock dose is 250µg/5ml. What volume of the drug should you give?

Drug Concentrations

Sometimes the stock dose of a drug may not be given as a weight in a particular volume, but rather as a percentage concentration of a solution.

For example, you may need to give a dose of a drug that is marked as 20% concentration. This percentage tells you the number of grams of that drug in 100ml of the solution.

For example, if a patient was prescribed 12g of a drug that was marked as 20% solution, you would work out the volume you give them as before using the prescribed dose as 12g and the stock dose as 20g/100ml.

This would be 12 ÷ 20 × 100 = 60ml.

Have a Go

800mg of a drug is prescribed. The drug is available in a 5% concentrate solution. What volume of the solution should you give to the patient?

Drug Strength Given as Ratio

As well as drug strengths expressed as a weight per volume or as a concentration, you may have a strength expressed as a ratio. This will usually be given in a format such as 1 in 10000.

A ratio like this tells you the number of grams of the drug in a number of millilitres of solution, so 1 in 10000 means that there is 1g of the drug in every 10000ml of the solution. It will sometimes help to convert these units to facilitate smaller doses. 1g/10000ml is the same as 1000mg/10000ml which is equivalent to 1mg/10ml.

As an example, consider a prescription of 45mg of a drug that is available in a 1 in 1000 ratio. This ratio means that there is 1g (1000mg) in every 1000ml of the drug, which means there is 1mg/ml. You can now work out what volume of the solution to give. $45 \div 1 \times 1 = 45$ml.

Have a Go

A patient has a 75mg prescription of a drug that is available in a 1 in 100 solution. What volume of the solution should you give?

Checking Answers

It is important to double-check the answers to your drug calculations. It is advisable to do the following to ensure the accuracy of your calculations:

- Make an estimate of what the dose should roughly be.

- Carry out the calculation on a calculator (twice).

- Check what a reasonable dose would be in a source such as 'BNF' or 'BNF for Children'.

If any of these cause doubt in the dosage calculated, check with a pharmacist or the person who made the prescription before administering the drug.

Practice Questions on Calculating Dosages

Question 1

200mg of a drug is prescribed. The stock dose is 50mg/5ml. What volume should be given?

Question 2

120mg of a drug is prescribed. The stock dose is 40mg/2ml. What volume should be given?

Question 3

350mg of a drug is prescribed. The stock dose is 200mg/10ml. What volume should be given?

Question 4

1.2g of a drug is prescribed. The stock dose is 400mg/5ml. What volume should be given?

Question 5

750µg of a drug is prescribed. The stock dose is 3mg/20ml. What volume should be given?

Question 6

5mg of a drug is prescribed. The stock dose is 500µg/6ml. What volume should be given?

Question 7

85mg of a drug is prescribed. The drug is available in a 1% concentrate solution. What volume of the solution should you give to the patient?

Question 8

200mg of a drug is prescribed. The drug is available in a 10% concentrate solution. What volume of the solution should you give to the patient?

Question 9

A patient has a 100mg prescription of a drug that is available in a 1 in 1000 solution. What volume of the solution should you give?

Question 10

A patient has a 25mg prescription of a drug that is available in a 1 in 10,000 solution. What volume of the solution should you give?

Solutions

Fully worked solutions to all of these questions can be accessed at www.mathsfornurses.com/calculatingdosages

Have a Go

1. 12ml

2. 30ml

3. 16ml

4. 7.5ml

Practice Questions

1. 20ml

2. 6ml

3. 17.5ml

4. 15ml

5. 5ml

6. 60ml

7. 8.5ml

8. 2ml

9. 100ml

10. 250ml

Oral Dosages

Tablets & Capsules

One of the most common ways of administering medicines is through tablets and capsules.

Often you will be given a prescription that states the total quantity of a drug to be given and you will need to work out how many tablets or capsules to administer to the patient to fulfil the prescription.

You will be able to find out the amount of the drug in each tablet or capsule, and to work out how many you need to give to the patient, divide the total amount of the drug that has been prescribed by the amount of the drug in each tablet or capsule.

For example, a doctor may prescribe 800mg of ibuprofen to be taken every 6 hours. If the tablets that are available are ibuprofen 200mg, this means that each tablet contains 200mg of ibuprofen, so the total amount of tablets that needs to be taken is 800 ÷ 200 = 4 tablets.

Number of Tablets = Prescribed Dose ÷ Dose in 1 Tablet

Have a Go

A patient is prescribed to take 20mg of citalopram daily. Citalopram 10mg tablets are available. How many tablets should the patient take each day?

Splitting Tablets

In some calculations, the prescribed dose may not work out to be a whole number of tablets.

If, for example, in the situation described above, the prescription had been for 500mg of ibuprofen to be taken every 6 hours (rather than 800mg) and the available tablets were still ibuprofen 200mg, then the amount of tablets required would be 500 ÷ 200 = 2.5 tablets.

When you get an answer like this, you need to check that it is appropriate to split a tablet or capsule. If you are not sure, ask the person who issued the prescription or a pharmacist before splitting the tablet.

Have a Go

A patient is prescribed to take 5mg of zafirlukast twice daily. Zafirlukast 20mg tablets are available. How many tablets should the patient be given for each dose?

Calculating Oral Dosage for Paediatrics*

When working with children or neonates, it is likely that the prescribed dose will be less than the amount contained in one tablet or capsule.

Depending on the particular proportion of a tablet or capsule that you need, you could split or crush a tablet or capsule (be sure to check that this is appropriate for the particular drug that you are administering).

To administer a particular portion of a tablet, crush the whole tablet thoroughly into a powder, and then ensure that the powder is fully dissolved into a particular quantity of water.

You can then calculate the volume of the solution to give using a method similar to the method outlined in the chapter on 'Calculating Dosages'.

For example, if each tablet contains 5mg of a drug, and your prescription instructs you to administer 2mg of the drug, you could crush the tablet and dissolve it in 10ml of water.

The amount of this solution that you would administer to the patient is $2 \div 5 \times 10 = 4$ml.

Have a Go

6mg of a drug is prescribed. The drug is available in 20mg tablets. If you were to crush one tablet and dissolve it in 5ml of water, what volume of the solution would you give to the patient?

Sometimes the amount of the solution that you are to administer may not work out as an exact amount (and in practice you cannot administer anything more precise than 0.01ml) so you will need to round your answer.

For example, a prescription is for 4mg of a drug that is available in 15ml tablets. If you were to crush one tablet and dissolve it in 10ml of water, the volume of the solution that you would need to administer is $4 \div 15 \times 10 = 2.666666...mL$

This decimal would keep recurring forever, so you need to round your answer to two decimal places to leave it with the most precise dose that you can administer. In this case, the volume of the solution would be 2.67ml.

Note – make sure that you check that the dose you give is close to the dose prescribed (it needs to be within 10% of the prescribed dose). Again, if you are unsure ask the person who made the prescription or a pharmacist.

Have a Go

A patient is prescribed 16mg of prednisone. A prednisone 30mg tablet is crushed and dissolved in 4ml of water. How much of the solution should be administered? Round your answer to an appropriate degree of accuracy.

Practice Questions on Oral Dosage (Adult)

Question 1

A patient is prescribed to take 10mg of diazepam twice a day. Diazepam 5mg tablets are available. How many tablets should the patient take for each dose?

Question 2

A patient is prescribed 120mg of orlistat three times per day. Orlistat 120mg tablets are available. How many tablets should the patient take for each dose?

Question 3

A patient is given a prescription for 2g of azithromycin. Azithromycin 250mg tablets are available. How many tablets should the patient take?

Question 4

A patient is prescribed 30mg of omeprazole. Omeprazole 20mg tablets are available. How many tablets should be taken?

Question 5

A patient is prescribed 160mg of ferrous sulphate. Ferrous sulphate is available in tablets that each contain 320mg of ferrous sulphate. How many tablets should the patient be given?

Practice Questions on Oral Dosage (Paediatric)*

Question 6

10mg of a drug is prescribed. The drug is available in 25mg tablets. If you were to crush one tablet and dissolve it in 5ml of water, what volume of the solution would you give to the patient?

Question 7

15mg of a drug is prescribed. The drug is available in 20mg tablets. If you were to crush one tablet and dissolve it in 4ml of water, what volume of the solution would you give to the patient?

Question 8

3mg of a drug is prescribed. The drug is available in 5mg tablets. If you were to crush one tablet and dissolve it in 10ml of water, what volume of the solution would you give to the patient?

Question 9

A patient is prescribed 10mg of a drug. A tablet containing 12mg of the drug is crushed and dissolved in 1ml of water. How much of the solution should be given to the patient?

Question 10

A patient is prescribed 2.5mg of olanzapine. Olanzapine 7.5mg tablets are available and one tablet is crushed and dissolved in 2ml of water. What volume of the solution should be given to the patient?

Solutions

Fully worked solutions to all of these questions can be accessed at www.mathsfornurses.com/oraldosages

Have a Go

1. 2

2. ¼

3. 1.5ml

4. 2.13ml

Practice Questions

1. 2

2. 1

3. 8

4. 1½

5. ½

6. 2ml

7. 3ml

8. 6ml

9. 0.83ml

10. 0.67ml

Intravenous Dosages

Another kind of calculation that you will need to be able to make is the dosage of a drug that is to be administered intravenously.

In this situation, you will usually have a drug that is already made up in a solution in a vial or ampoule.

For example, you may have a drug that is available in 50mg in 5ml ampoules. This means that in each ampoule there is 50mg of the drug dissolved in 5ml of the solution.

If you were administering a prescription of 200mg, then this is the same as four of the ampoules so you would need to administer 20ml of the solution.

Divide the amount of drug prescribed by the amount of drug in the ampoule or vial and multiply the answer by the total volume of the ampoule or vial.

IV Dose = Prescribed Dose ÷ Amount of Drug in Ampoule × Volume in Ampoule

---

In the example above, this would mean that your calculation would be 200 ÷ 50 × 5 = 20ml (as before).

As another example, think of a patient who had been prescribed 2mg of a drug that is available in 500µg in 100ml vials.

In this situation, the measurements have been given in different units so one of them will need to be converted. To avoid working with decimals it will be best to convert the 2mg into micrograms, so this will be 2,000µg.

Now substitute these numbers into your formula. 2,000 ÷ 500 x 100 = 400ml.

Have a Go

A patient is prescribed 12mg of a drug that is available in 2mg in 50ml ampoules. How much of the solution should be administered?

International Units

A lot of the calculations that you perform will be with drugs that are measured in grams, milligrams or micrograms. However, it also possible that you may encounter certain drugs that are measured in International Units.

When working with International Units, both the prescribed dose and the amount of drug in the ampoule should be given in International Units (if not, check with the person who made the prescription or a pharmacist). You can carry out the calculation exactly as before.

For example, a patient may be prescribed 3 million International Units of colistemethate sodium, and the colistemethate sodium may be available in 1 million International Units in 20ml vials.

The volume of the solution that you would administer is worked out using the formula above. 3,000,000 ÷ 1,000,000 × 20 = 60ml.

Have a Go

A patient is prescribed 60 International Units of actrapid, which is available in 400 International Units in 10ml vials. How much of the solution should be administered to the patient?

Calculating Intravenous Dosage for Paediatrics*

When preparing intravenous drugs for children and neonates, there are a few extra factors to take into account. The amount of solution administered will need to take into account the child's fluid allowances. The doses may be particularly small and precision is crucial. It is good practice to check these calculations thoroughly and if there is any doubt to also have the calculation checked by somebody else independently

A further factor to consider is the displacement value of the drug. When the drug is in the form of a powder to be dissolved in a solution with fluid the drug itself will add to the overall volume of the solution. This must be taken into account when working out how much fluid to add.

For example, a drug may be in the form of a powder and may need to be prepared as a solution containing 100mg in 10ml of the solution. The drug may be available in 100mg vials that have a displacement value of 0.5ml. This means that to make up a total of 10ml, you would need to add 9.5ml of the fluid for the solution.

> ## Amount of Fluid to Add = Total Fluid Needed – Displacement Value

Have a Go

A drug is available as a 150mg vial that has a displacement value of 0.1ml and needs to be made up as a solution containing 150mg in 5ml. How much fluid would you need to add to the solution?

Another consideration when calculating dosage for infants and neonates is that the dose is rarely expressed as a fixed quantity and is more frequently given as a quantity per kilogram. Calculations of this kind are the topic of the next chapter.

Practice Questions on Intravenous Dosage (Adult)

Question 1

A patient is prescribed 8mg of a drug that is available in 4mg in 10ml ampoules. How much of the solution should be administered?

Question 2

A patient is prescribed 60mg of a drug that is available in 15mg in 100ml ampoules. How much of the solution should be administered?

Question 3

A patient is prescribed 250mg of a drug that is available in 100mg in 50ml ampoules. How much of the solution should be administered?

Question 4

A patient is prescribed 500μg of a drug that is available in 2mg in 20ml ampoules. How much of the solution should be administered?

Question 5

A patient is prescribed 500,000 International Units of colomycin, which is available in 1 million International Units in 80ml ampoules. How much of the solution should be administered to the patient?

Question 6

A patient is prescribed 32 million International Units of interferon beta-1b, which is available in 4 million International Units in 20ml ampoules. How much of the solution should be administered to the patient?

Question 7

A patient is prescribed 4000 International Units of enoxaparin sodium, which is available in 2000 International Units in 0.2ml ampoules. How much of the solution should be administered to the patient?

Practice Questions on Intravenous Dosage (Paediatric)*

Question 8

A drug is available as a 100mg vial that has a displacement value of 1ml and needs to be made up as a solution containing 100mg in 20ml. How much fluid would you need to add to the solution?

Question 9

A drug is available as a 20mg vial that has a displacement value of 0.2ml and needs to be made up as a solution containing 20mg in 5ml. How much fluid would you need to add to the solution?

Question 10

A drug is available as a 50mg vial that has a displacement value of 0.5ml and needs to be made up as a solution containing 50mg in 100ml. How much fluid would you need to add to the solution?

Solutions

Fully worked solutions to all of these questions can be accessed at www.mathsfornurses.com/intravenousdosages

Have a Go

1. 300ml
2. 1.5ml
3. 4.9ml

Practice Questions

1. 20ml
2. 400ml
3. 125ml
4. 5ml
5. 40ml
6. 160ml
7. 0.4ml
8. 19ml
9. 4.8ml
10. 99.5ml

Dosage Per Weight*

So far we have considered situations in which a specific quantity of a drug is prescribed. It is often the case (especially in paediatrics, though sometimes in adult medicine too) that the dosage prescribed will not be the total dose but will depend on the weight of a patient.

For example, if the prescribed dose is 3mg/kg it means that you will need to administer 3 milligrams of the drug for every kilogram of the patient's weight. You can calculate the required dose by multiplying the patient's weight in kilograms by 3. If this dose were prescribed to a patient weighing 12kg, the dose you would need to give is 12 × 3 = 36mg.

As another example, a patient who weighs 55kg may be prescribed 2mg/kg of a drug. The dose that you would need to give to this patient is 55 × 2 = 110mg.

Have a Go

A patient who weighs 24kg is prescribed 5mg/kg of a drug. What is the total dosage that you will need to administer?

You will often encounter a prescription given per weight as part of another drug calculation. When this happens, start by working out the total dose and then carry out your calculation as before.

For example, a patient who weighs 30kg may be prescribed 1.5mg/kg of a drug that is available with a stock dose of 3mg/10ml.

To work out the total volume that you need to administer, start by working out the required dose. 1.5 × 30 = 45mg. The problem now becomes a drug calculation where you want to give 45mg of a drug that has a stock dose of 3mg/10ml. You can work this out as described in the chapter on 'Calculating Dosages'. 45 ÷ 3 × 10 = 150ml.

Have a Go

A patient who weighs 56kg is prescribed 2.5mg/kg of a drug that is available with a stock dose of 7mg/5ml. What is the total volume of the solution that you will need to administer?

Unit Conversions

When calculating dosage per weight you will often be in situations where you need to convert units to make your calculation. The conversions that you are most likely to need in this context are 1mg = 1000µg and 1g = 1000mg (for more on how to convert between different units, see chapter on 'Converting Measurements').

For example, a patient who weighs 20kg may be prescribed 650µg/kg of a drug that is available with a stock dose of 2mg/5ml.

In this example, when you work out the prescribed dose, you will get 20 × 650 = 13000µg. The stock dose, however, is measured in **milligrams** per millilitre, so you will need to convert the required dose into milligrams too. 13000µg = 13mg. You can then proceed as before. 13 ÷ 2 x 5 = 32.5ml.

Have a Go

A patient who weighs 60kg is prescribed 40mg/kg of a drug that is available with a stock dose of 1g/100ml. What is the total volume of the solution that you will need to administer?

Dose Per Surface Area

In some contexts (for example cancer treatments), drugs are calculated per surface area rather than per volume. For example, a dose may be stated as $1.5mg/m^2$, which means that 1.5mg of the drug should be administered for each metre squared of the patient's surface area.

If a patient has a body surface area of $2m^2$, the amount of the drug given should be 1.5 × 2 = $3m^2$.

Again, this could come up as part of another drug calculation question. For example, if the prescription is for $0.8mg/m^2$ and the patient has a body surface area of $0.5m^2$ and the drug is available with a stock dose of 1mg/5ml, you would start by working out the total dose to be given. 0.8 × 0.5 = 0.4mg. Now calculate the volume of the solution to administer as before. 0.4 ÷ 1 × 5 = 2ml

Have a Go

A patient with a body surface area of $1.6m^2$ is prescribed $5mg/m^2$ of a drug that is available with a stock dose of 10mg/ml. What volume of the solution should you administer?

Calculating Surface Area

You may need to a work out a dosage based on surface area for a patient for whom you do not know their body surface area.

There are several different calculations that you can use to estimate a patient's surface area based on their weight and/or height. The most commonly used of these calculations is Mosteller's Formula.

$$\text{Body Surface Area} = \sqrt{\frac{W \times H}{3600}}$$

In this formula, W refers to the weight of the patient in kilograms and H refers to the patient's height in centimetres. To estimate the surface area you need to multiply together the weight and the height, divide the answer by 3600 and then square root this answer.

For example, you could estimate the surface area of a woman with height 160cm and weight 55km. $160 \times 55 = 8800 \div 3600 = 2.44$. $\sqrt{2.44} = 1.56m^2$.

In order to check that your answers are realistic, you can compare them to the average surface areas below:

- Neonate: $0.25m^2$
- Child (Age 2): $0.5m^2$
- Child (Age 10): $1.14m^2$
- Adult Female: $1.6m^2$
- Adult Male: $1.9m^2$

Your surface area may be slightly higher or lower than the average, but if it is on a completely different order of magnitude (e.g. if your answer is $100m^2$) then you known that a mistake has been made.

In the example above, the surface area of a woman has been calculated to be $1.56m^2$. The average surface area for women is $1.6m^2$, which is close to the surface area that has been calculated so you can be confident that the calculation has been made accurately.

You may need to use this method of calculating body surface area as part of a calculation. For example, if a child of age 2 who is 89cm tall and weighs 13kg is prescribed $8mg/m^2$ of a drug that is available with a stock dose of 2mg/5ml you can work out the volume of the solution to give.

First work out the surface area of the patient using Mosteller's formula. 89 × 13 = 1157 ÷ 3600 = 0.32. √0.32 = 0.57m². As the average surface area of a 2 year old is 0.5m² you can be confident in this calculation. The dosage required is 8mg × 0.57 = 4.54mg. Now work out how much of the solution to give. 4.54 ÷ 2 × 5 = 11.4ml.

Have a Go

A man with a height of 185cm and weight 73kg is prescribed 3.5mg/m² of a drug that is available with a stock dose of 5mg/10ml. What volume of the solution should you administer?

Practice Questions on Dosage Per Weight

Question 1

A patient weighing 35kg is prescribed a dose of 4mg/kg. What dose should be given?

Question 2

A patient weighing 62kg is prescribed a dose of 2.5mg/kg. What dose should be given?

Question 3

A patient weighing 14kg is prescribed a dose of 6mg/kg of a drug with a stock dose of 4mg/10ml. What volume of the solution should be administered?

Question 4

A patient weighing 8kg is prescribed a dose of 15mg/kg of a drug that is available in 20mg in 10ml ampoules. How much of the solution should be administered?

Question 5

A patient weighing 25kg is prescribed 400µg/kg of a drug that is available in 5mg tablets. How many tablets should be taken?

Question 6

A patient weighing 60kg is prescribed 50mg/kg of a drug that is available in 0.5g/200ml solution. How much of the solution should be administered?

Question 7

A patient with body surface area of $1.7m^2$ is prescribed $3mg/m^2$ of a drug that is available in a stock dose of 1mg/2ml. How much of the solution should be administered?

Question 8

A patient with a surface area of $1.3m^2$ is prescribed $1000 units/m^2$ of a drug that is available in a stock dose of 100 units/5ml. What volume of the solution should be administered?

Question 9

A woman with a height of 145cm and weight 59kg is prescribed $2.6mg/m^2$ of a drug that is available with a stock dose of 2mg/5ml. What volume of the solution should you administer?

Question 10

A new-born baby with a height of 48cm and weight 2.6kg is prescribed $1.2mg/m^2$ of a drug that is available with a stock dose of 1mg/10ml. What volume of the solution should you administer?

Solutions

Fully worked solutions to all of these questions can be accessed at www.mathsfornurses.com/dosageperweight

Have a Go

1. 120mg

2. 100ml

3. 240ml

4. 0.8ml

5. 13.6ml

Practice Questions

1. 140mg

2. 155mg

3. 210ml

4. 60ml

5. 2

6. 1.2L

7. 10.2ml

8. 65ml

9. 10ml

10. 2.3ml

Multiple Doses

A prescription may be given that specifies that more than one dose of a medicine should be administered. For example, a patient may be prescribed 15mg of a drug three times a day. In order to work out the total amount of the drug given, multiply the size of an individual dose by the number of doses that will be given. In this case, the total amount of the drug given each day will be 3 × 15mg = 45mg.

Have a Go

What is the total amount that will be administered to a patient who is prescribed 75mg of a drug 4 times per day?

In order to calculate the total dosage, you need to know the number of doses that will be given. In the examples above you are told this information in the question, but sometimes you will need to work it out.

For example, you may know that a patient is given 30mg of a drug every 4 hours. If you want to work out how much of the drug is administered in a 24-hour period, you would need to work out how many 4-hour periods make up the full 24-hours. You can do this by dividing 24 by 4, so the dose will be given 6 times. You can then work out 6 × 30mg which makes a total of 180mg.

As another example, a patient may be prescribed 50mg of a drug, twice a day for a week. The total amount of the drug they will be given over the week can be calculated. Start by working out the total number of doses. 2 doses a day for 7 days makes a total of 2 × 7 = 14 doses. The total amount of the drug given will be 14 × 50mg = 700mg.

Have a Go

A patient is prescribed 2.5mg of a drug every 2 hours. How much of the drug will be administered over a 12-hour period?

Often you will need to work out these dosages as part of other drug calculation questions.

For example, if a patient is prescribed 40mg of a drug 3 times per day and the drug is available in 10mg tablets, you may want to work out the total number of tablets the patient will be given each day.

Start by working out how many tablets will be given in each dose. 40mg ÷ 10mg = 4 tablets. Because this dose needs to be given 3 times per day, the total number of tablets in a day will be 3 × 4 = 12.

As another example, a patient weighing 42kg is prescribed 8mg/kg twice per day. The stock dose of the drug is 20mg/5ml. Work out how much of the solution will be administered over a 24-hour period.

Again, start by working out a single dose. 42 × 8 = 336mg. The volume administered for this dose is 336 ÷ 20 × 5 = 84ml. Because this dose is given twice per day, the total volume administered in 24 hours is 84ml × 2 = 168ml.

Have a Go

A patient is prescribed 16mg of a drug every 3 hours. The drug is available in a 2mg/10ml solution. How much of the solution should be given over a 24-hour period?

Individual Doses

You may also need to make these calculations in reverse. If a patient is prescribed 200mg of a drug over a 24-hour period, to be split into four equal doses, then to find the size of each dose you would need to divide 200 by 4, so each dose would be 50mg.

Have a Go

A patient is prescribed a total of 60mg of a drug to be taken over a 24-hour period in equal doses every 4 hours. What size should each dose be?

Again, this may be in the context of other drug calculations. For example, a patient is prescribed 56mg of a drug to be given over a week with tablets to be taken each morning and evening. 2mg tablets are available. How many tablets should each dose be?

Start by working out a single prescribed dose. There will be a total of 7 × 2 = 14 doses, so each dose will be 56mg ÷ 14 = 4mg. Because each tablet is 2mg, the number of tablets required is 4mg ÷ 2mg = 2.

Have a Go

A patient weighing 24kg is prescribed 500µg/kg of a drug, to be given in 4 equal doses. The drug is available with a stock dose of 1mg/10ml. How much of the volume should be administered for each dose?

Important Abbreviations

Sometimes a prescription to give a dose more than once will be written using shorthand. It is important to know the meaning of the following terms (if you are unsure of the meaning of anything you see on a prescription, check with a pharmacist or the person who wrote the prescription before administering the medicine).

- **b.d.s. (or b.i.d. or just bd)** – twice per day
- **t.d.s. (or t.i.d. or just td)** – three times per day
- **q.d.s. (or q.i.d. or just qd)** – four times per day
- **q.h.** – every hour
- **q.2.h.** – every 2 hours (q.3.h. means every 3 hours and so on).

For example, a patient who is prescribed 30mg of a drug t.d.s. will need to be given 30mg × 3 = 90mg over the course of a day.

Have a Go

A patient is prescribed 45mg of a drug q.d.s. The drug is available with a stock dose of 4mg/5ml. How much of the solution should be administered over a 24-hour period?

Practice Questions on Multiple Doses

Question 1

A patient is prescribed 125mg of a drug to be taken every 4 hours. How much of the drug will be given over 24 hours?

Question 2

A patient is prescribed 15mg of a medicine three times per day for a week. What is the total amount of the medicine prescribed?

Question 3

A patient who weighs 55kg is prescribed 1mg/kg of a drug four times per day. The drug is available with a stock dose of 5mg/20ml. What volume of the solution will need to be prepared for a 24-hour period?

Question 4

A patient is prescribed 25mg of a drug every 3 hours. The stock dose is 4mg/10ml. How much of the solution will be required over the course of a day?

Question 5

A patient is prescribed 250mg of a drug to be taken in four equal doses. What is the size of each dose?

Question 6

A patient is prescribed 150mg of a drug to be taken over a 12-hour period in equal doses every 2 hours. How much should be given in each dose?

Question 7

A patient is prescribed a total of 120mg of a drug to be taken over a 24-hour period in four equal doses. The drug is available with a stock dose of 5mg/5ml. What volume of the solution should be administered for each dose?

Question 8

A patient with a weight of 15kg is prescribed a 600μg/kg of a drug to be taken over a 24 hours period in three equal doses. The drug is available with a stock dose of 4mg/20ml. How much of the solution should be administered for each dose?

Question 9

A patient is prescribed 35mg of a drug b.d.s. How much of the drug will he be given in a day?

Question 10

A patient is prescribed 40mg of a drug t.d.s. The drug is available with a stock dose of 1mg/10ml. How much of the solution should be prepared for a 24-hour period?

Solutions

Fully worked solutions to all of these questions can be accessed at www.mathsfornurses.com/multipledoses

Have a Go

1. 300mg

2. 15mg

3. 640ml

4. 10mg

5. 30ml

6. 225ml

Practice Questions

1. 750mg

2. 315mg

3. 880ml

4. 500ml

5. 62.5mg

6. 25mg

7. 30ml

8. 15ml

9. 70mg

10. 1.2L

Infusion Rates

Drip Rates

Fluids that are delivered intravenously are controlled by setting an administration device to a particular rate of infusion (also known as a drip rate). The drip rate tells you how many drops per minute of the solution should be administered.

To work out the drip rate that the device should be set to, you need to first work out the total number of drops to be administered. You will usually be provided with a basic number of drops per ml that will be administered (this will often be 20 drops per ml for a clear infusion fluid or 15ml for blood). Multiply this number by the total volume in ml that you need to administer.

Once you have worked out the total number of drops that you need to administer, divide this by the amount of time (in minutes) that the drug will be administered for.

For example, to administer 300ml of 0.9% sodium chloride injection fluid, which is delivered at 20 drops per ml, over a 2-hour period, first work out the total number of drops required. 300 × 20 = 6000. The time in minutes is 2 × 60 = 120, so the drip rate will be 6000 ÷ 120 = 50 drops per minute.

Have a Go

> What flow rate should you set to administer 500ml of a fluid that is delivered at 20 drops per ml over a 3-hour period?

Sometimes you will need to calculate a drip rate in the context of another drug calculation. For example, what is the required drip rate to administer a 30mg dose over 60 minutes, if a drug is available in an infusion fluid with a stock dose 2 mg/5ml that is delivered at 20 drops per ml?

First calculate the total volume of the solution required. 30 ÷ 2 × 5 = 75ml. Next, work out the number of drops that will be required to deliver this volume. 75 × 20 = 1500ml. Finally, work out the drip rate. 1500 ÷ 60 = 25 drips per minute.

Have a Go

A patient is prescribed 80mg of a drug to be delivered over 4 hours. The drug is available with a stock dose of 1mg/5ml that is delivered at 20 drops per ml. What should the drip rate be set at?

In some situations, you will already know the required drip rate and need to work out the amount of time required to administer the total volume.

For example, blood is usually delivered at 15 drips per ml. If you want to administer 600ml of blood at a drip rate of 30 drips per minute, you can work out how long you should administer the blood for.

As before, start by working out the total number of drops required. 600 × 15 = 9000. You can work out the number of minutes by dividing the number of drops by the drip rate. 9000 ÷ 30 = 300, so you need to administer blood for 300 minutes, which is 5 hours.

Have a Go

0.9 Sodium Chloride fluid is delivered at 20 drips per ml. How long will it take to administer 1 litre of 0.9 Sodium Chloride if the drip rate is set to 80 drops per minute?

Infusion Devices

When a drug is administered by an infusion device, the rate of infusion is not measured by counting the rate of drips but rather by directly monitoring how much of the drug is being administered over a period of time. This may be tracked either according to the amount of the drug (for example 10mg per hour) or the volume of fluid (for example 10ml per minute).

For example, if you need to administer 300ml of a solution over a period of 5 hours, then you would find your infusion rate in ml per hour by dividing the total volume by the time. 300 ÷ 5 = 60ml/hour.

Similarly, to deliver 3g of a drug over a 24 hour period, you would first convert the 3g into 3000mg, then divide by the time frame so the infusion rate will be 3000 ÷ 24 = 125mg/hour.

Have a Go

What infusion rate (in millilitres per hour) would be required to deliver 180ml of a fluid over 1 hour, 30 minutes?

Syringe Drivers

When a drug is delivered by a syringe driver, the syringe is pushed forward at a specified rate to administer the drug.

To use a syringe driver, first prepare the prescribed solution in the syringe and measure the distance that the plunger will need to travel in the syringe (known as the stroke length). This stroke length will vary according to the type of syringe that is being used.

The infusion rate will either be set in mm per hour or mm per day (note – it is important to check carefully which of these is being used).

To work out this rate, divide the total stroke length by the time.

For example, a syringe with stroke length 54mm that is measured in mm per hour needs to be delivered over 6 hours. The required rate will be 54 ÷ 6 = 9mm per hour.

Similarly, a syringe with stroke length 60mm that is measured in mm per day needs to be delivered over 48 hours. Convert 48 hours into 2 days, so the rate will be 60 ÷ 2 = 30 mm per day.

Have a Go

A syringe with stroke length 72mm needs to be delivered over 1 day. What rate should the syringe be set to in mm per hour?

Practice Questions on Infusion Rates

Question 1

What flow rate should you set to administer 600ml of a fluid that is delivered at 20 drops per ml over an 8-hour period?

Question 2

If you want to administer 400ml of blood at 15 drops per ml over a 2-hour period, what drip rate would you need to set?

Question 3

A patient is prescribed 125mg of a drug to be delivered over 4 hours. The drug is available with a stock dose of 20mg/80ml that is delivered at 20 drops per ml. What should the drip rate be set at?

Question 4

A patient is prescribed 80mg of a drug to be delivered over 6 hours. The drug is available with a stock dose of 1mg/10ml that is delivered at 30 drops per ml. What should the drip rate be set at?

Question 5

An infusion fluid is delivered at 20 drips per ml. How long will it take to administer 600ml of the fluid if the drip rate is set to 40 drops per minute?

Question 6

An infusion fluid is delivered at 20 drips per ml. How long will it take to deliver 30mg of a drug infused in a solution with stock dose 10mg/15ml if the drip rate is set to 30 drips per minute?

Question 7

What infusion rate (in millilitres per hour) would be required to deliver 400ml of a fluid over 2 hours, 30 minutes?

Question 8

What infusion rate (in millilitres per minute) would be required to deliver 15mg of a drug infused in a solution with stock dose 1mg/5ml over 30 minutes?

Question 9

A syringe with stroke length 48mm needs to be delivered over 8 hours. What rate should the syringe be set to in mm per hour?

Question 10

A syringe with stroke length 60mm needs to be delivered over 36 hours. What rate should the syringe be set to in mm per day?

Solutions

Fully worked solutions to all of these questions can be accessed at www.mathsfornurses.com/infusionrates

Have a Go

1. 56 drops per minute

2. 33 drops per minute

3. 4 hours, 10 minutes

4. 120ml per hour

5. 3mm per hour

Practice Questions

1. 25 drops per minute

2. 50 drops per minute

3. 42 drops per minute

4. 67 drops per minute

5. 5 hours

6. 30 minutes

7. 160 millilitres per hour

8. 2.5 millilitres per minute

9. 6 millimetres per hour

10. 40 millimetres per day

Fluid Balance*

In order for metabolic processes to function correctly, it is important that fluid levels are monitored in a patient.

Fluid Balance Charts

One of the most common ways of monitoring fluids is using a fluid balance chart, as shown in the diagram below.

TIME	INPUT					OUTPUT		
	Oral Input	Volume	IV Input	Volume	Running Total	Urine	Other	Running Total
00:00								
01:00								
02:00								
03:00								
04:00								
05:00								
06:00								
07:00								
08:00			0.9% Saline	1200ml	1200ml			
09:00	Water	200ml			1400ml			
10:00						200ml		200ml
11:00							350ml	550ml
12:00	Juice	150ml			1550ml			
13:00						500ml		1050ml
14:00	Water	100ml			1650ml			
15:00						150ml		1200ml
16:00								
17:00							200ml	1400ml
18:00	Water	250ml			1900ml			
19:00						400ml		1800ml
20:00								
21:00								
22:00	Tea	100ml			2000ml			
23:00						100ml		1900ml
Total		800ml		1200ml	2000ml	1350ml	550ml	1900ml

This table keeps track of the fluid input and output of the patient hour-by-hour. On this table, fluid input is categorised as oral or intravenous, with space to record the type of the input and the volume (fluid balance charts can vary slightly and you may come across them categorised slightly differently).

For example, this table shows that the first fluid input was 1200ml of 0.9% saline, administered intravenously at 08:00. After this was a drink of 200ml of water at 09:00, 150ml of juice at 12:00, 100ml of water at 14:00, 250ml of water at 18:00 and finally 100ml of tea at 22:00.

As well as recording the volumes of each individual input, the table shows a running total of all inputs for the day. At 08:00, the only input is the 1200ml of saline, so this is recorded as the running total. At 09:00, the 200ml is added to the running total, which now becomes 1400ml. Each time a new input is recorded on the table, this volume is added to the running total.

In the right-hand section of the table, the outputs are recorded. Here they are categorised as urine and other (vomit, bowels, drain etc.) but again they may sometimes be categorised slightly differently. The outputs are recorded by writing down the volume of the output at the time it happened. In this case, the first output was 200ml of urine at 10:00, and then 350ml of an 'other' output at 11:00. These were followed by 500ml of urine at 13:00, 150ml of urine at 15:00, 200ml of 'other' at 17:00, 400ml of urine at 19:00 and finally 100ml of urine at 23:00. Again, a running total is kept, and the overall totals are recorded at the bottom of the fluid table. In this case the patient took in 2000ml of fluid in the day and their total output was 1900ml.

If you need to work out the total fluid input of a patient for a day, add together all of the individual inputs, and to work out the total output for the day, add together the individual outputs.

Have a Go

Over a 24-hour period, Lisa's fluid inputs are 900ml, 350ml, 200ml, 120ml and 75ml. Her fluid outputs are 500ml, 400ml, 320ml, 180ml and 150ml. Work out Lisa's total fluid input and output.

Have a Go

On the fluid balance table below, fill in the running totals and work out the total input and output.

TIME	INPUT					OUTPUT		
	Oral Input	Volume	IV Input	Volume	Running Total	Urine	Other	Running Total
00:00								
01:00								
02:00			0.9% Saline	800ml				
03:00								
04:00								
05:00								
06:00						250ml		
07:00								
08:00								
09:00	Water	100ml					150ml	
10:00								
11:00							200ml	
12:00			0.9% Saline	800ml				
13:00						300ml		
14:00								
15:00	Water	250ml				250ml		
16:00								
17:00								
18:00	Juice	100ml						
19:00								
20:00						500ml		
21:00	Water	150ml						
22:00								
23:00						150ml		
Total								

Maintenance Fluid Rates*

In order to maintain healthy fluid levels in a patient, you need to work out how much fluid that they actually need. This is called the maintenance fluid rate, and it will depend on the weight of the patient.

The formula used will be different for adults and for children.

For adults, the recommended fluid intake is 25-35ml/kg/day (though this may vary – particularly if the patient is losing fluid).

For example, if a patient weighs 80kg, then the amount of the fluid that they should take in will be between 25 × 80 = 2000ml (or 2L) and 35 × 80 = 2800ml (or 2.8L).

Have a Go

How much fluid should an adult patient weighing 55kg take in over 24 hours?

In paediatric medicine, the maintenance fluid rate is 100ml/kg for the first 10kg of the patient's weight, 50ml/kg for the next 10kg, and 20ml/kg thereafter.

For example, work out the maintenance fluid required for a child who weighs 24kg. The first 10kg will need 10 × 100 = 1000ml. The next 10kg will need 10 × 50 = 500ml and the final 4kg will need 4 × 20 = 80ml, so the total fluid required will be 1580ml.

Have a Go?

How much fluid should a child weighing 18kg take in over 24 hours?

Practice Questions on Fluid Balance

Over a 24-hour period, Joshua's fluid inputs are 600ml, 500ml, 240ml, 200ml and 135ml. His fluid outputs are 650ml, 475ml, 190ml, 65ml and 50ml.

Question 1

What is Joshua's total fluid input?

Question 2

What is Joshua's total fluid output?

The fluid balance table below shows the fluid input and output for Mrs Watson over a 24-hour period.

TIME	INPUT					OUTPUT		
	Oral Input	Volume	IV Input	Volume	Running Total	Urine	Other	Running Total
00:00								
01:00								
02:00								
03:00								
04:00								
05:00								
06:00			0.9% Saline	500ml				
07:00							200ml	
08:00								
09:00							400ml	
10:00			0.9% Saline	500ml				
11:00						350ml		
12:00								
13:00								
14:00			0.9% Saline	500ml				
15:00						250ml		
16:00								
17:00							300ml	
18:00			0.9% Saline	500ml				
19:00								
20:00	Water	150ml				400ml		
21:00								
22:00								
23:00								
Total								

Question 3

What was Mrs Watson's total fluid input?

Question 4

What was Mrs Watson's total fluid output?

The fluid balance table below shows the fluid input and output for Mr Johnson over a 24-hour period.

TIME	INPUT					OUTPUT		
	Oral Input	Volume	IV Input	Volume	Running Total	Urine	Other	Running Total
00:00								
01:00								
02:00								
03:00								
04:00								
05:00								
06:00							250ml	
07:00								
08:00								
09:00	Water	400ml					250ml	
10:00								
11:00	Tea	150ml						
12:00							250ml	
13:00	Milk	200ml				100ml		
14:00								
15:00							250ml	
16:00	Water	300ml						
17:00								
18:00	Juice	150ml					250ml	
19:00								
20:00								
21:00	Water	150ml				150ml		
22:00								
23:00								
Total								

Question 5

What was Mr Johnson's total fluid input?

Question 6

What was Mr Johnson's total fluid output?

Question 7

How much fluid should an adult patient weighing 62kg take in over 24 hours?

Question 8

How much fluid should an adult patient weighing 96kg take in over 24 hours?

Question 9

How much fluid should a child weighing 32kg take in over 24 hours?

Question 10

How much fluid should a child weighing 6kg take in over 24 hours?

Solutions

Fully worked solutions to all of these questions can be accessed at www.mathsfornurses.com/fluidbalance

Have a Go

1. Input – 1645ml, Output – 1550ml

2. Input – 2200ml, Output – 1800ml

3. Between 1375ml and 1925ml

4. 1400ml

Practice Questions

1. 1675ml

2. 1430ml

3. 2150ml

4. 1900ml

5. 1350ml

6. 1500ml

7. Between 1550ml and 2170ml

8. Between 2400ml and 3360ml

9. 1740ml

10. 600ml

Burns

When a patient has suffered second- or third-degree burns, then their fluid requirements over the first 24-hours can be calculated using the Parkland Formula. This formula takes into account both the weight of the patient and the percentage of their body that is covered with burns.

Fluid Requirement = 4 × Mass × Percentage Burns

Use this formula to work out the fluid requirement in millilitres, by multiplying the weight in kilograms by 4 and multiplying this answer by the percentage of the body that is covered with burns.

For example, if a patient weighs 60kg and 15% of their body is covered with burns, their fluid requirement will be 4 × 60 × 15 = 3600ml.

Half of this will be delivered over the first 8 hours after the burn and the other half will be delivered in the next 16 hours after that.

Have a Go?

How much fluid will be required in the first 24 hours for a patient weighing 85kg who has 30% of his body covered with burns?

To estimate the percentage of the body that has been covered with burns, you can use the Wallace rule – 9% of the total surface area is in each arm, 18% in each leg, 18% for the front of the torso, 18% for the back of the torso, 9% for the head and 1% for the perineum. You can add up the relevant percentages to find the total percentage of the body surface area that has suffered burns (or if burns are only partial on one of these areas of the body, then adjust the percentage accordingly).

Practice Questions on Burns

Question 1

How much fluid will be required in the first 24 hours for a patient weighing 72kg who has 20% of his body covered with burns?

Question 2

How much fluid will be required in the first 24 hours for a patient weighing 56kg who has 15% of her body covered with burns?

Question 3

How much fluid will be required in the first 24 hours for a patient weighing 64kg who has 24% of his body covered with burns?

Question 4

How much fluid will be required in the first 24 hours for a patient weighing 90kg who has 13% of his body covered with burns?

Question 5

How much fluid will be required in the first 24 hours for a patient weighing 47kg who has 45% of her body covered with burns?

Solutions

Fully worked solutions to all of these questions can be accessed at www.mathsfornurses.com/burns

Have a Go

1. 10200ml

Practice Questions

1. 5760ml

2. 3360ml

3. 6144ml

4. 4680ml

5. 8460ml

Practice Test E

Question 1

A patient is prescribed 75mg of a drug to be taken in six equal doses. What is the size of each dose?

Question 2

A patient is prescribed to take 800mg of ibuprofen three times per day. How many ibuprofen 200mg tablets should be taken for each dose?

Question 3

Lidocaine is available in a 0.1% solution. How much of the solution should be given if 5mg of Lidocaine are prescribed?

Question 4

What flow rate should you set to administer 750ml of a fluid that is delivered at 20 drops per ml over a 4-hour period?

Question 5

A drug is available as a 50mg vial that has a displacement value of 4ml and needs to be made up as a solution containing 50mg in 100ml. How much fluid would you need to add to the solution?

Question 6

How much fluid will be required in the first 24 hours for a patient weighing 35kg who has 16% of his body covered with burns?

Question 7

A patient with a surface area of 1.6m² is prescribed 500 units/m² of a drug that is available in a stock dose of 200 units/5ml. What volume of the solution should be administered?

Question 8

Here is the fluid balance chart for a patient's fluid input and output over a 24-hour period.

TIME	Oral Input	Volume	IV Input	Volume	Running Total	Urine	Other	Running Total
	INPUT					**OUTPUT**		
00:00								
01:00								
02:00								
03:00								
04:00								
05:00								
06:00	Water	150ml						
07:00						350ml		
08:00								
09:00			0.9% Saline	800ml				
10:00							250ml	
11:00								
12:00	Water	300ml						
13:00						100ml		
14:00								
15:00	Tea	200ml						
16:00						400ml		
17:00								
18:00	Juice	250ml						
19:00								
20:00						100ml		
21:00	Water	50ml						
22:00								
23:00						100ml		
Total								

Work out his total fluid input and output.

Question 9

A patient is prescribed 100mg of a drug q.d.s. The drug is available with a stock dose of 10mg/10ml. How much of the solution should be prepared for a 24-hour period?

Question 10

A patient is prescribed 500µg of adrenaline. The adrenaline is available with a stock dose of 1mg/2ml. How much adrenaline should be administered?

Question 11

8mg of a drug is prescribed to a child. The drug is available in 20mg tablets. If you were to crush one tablet and dissolve it in 50ml of water, what volume of the solution would you give to the patient?

Question 12

What infusion rate (in millilitres per minute) would be required to administer 250mg of a drug infused in a solution with stock dose 2mg/5ml over 2 hours?

Solutions

Worked solutions to test E can be accessed at www.mathsfornurses.com/practicetestse-h

1. 12.5mg

2. 4

3. 5ml

4. 63 drops per minute

5. 96ml

6. 2240ml

7. 20ml

8. Input – 1750ml, Output – 1300ml

9. 400ml

10. 1ml

11. 20ml

12. 5.2ml/min

Practice Test F

Question 1

A patient in prescribed 700µg of a drug that is available in 5mg in 100ml ampoules. How much of the solution should be administered?

Question 2

A patient is prescribed 3mg of dexamethasone. The drug is available in a solution of 0.5mg in 5ml. What volume of the solution should be administered?

Question 3

A man with a height of 170cm and weight 80kg is prescribed $1.5mg/m^2$ of a drug that is available with a stock dose of 5mg/20ml. What volume of the solution should be given?

Question 4

A patient who weighs 36kg is prescribed 1.5mg/kg of a drug three times per day. The drug is available with a stock dose of 2mg/5ml. What volume of the solution will need to be prepared for a 24-hour period?

Question 5

How much fluid should an adult patient weighing 74kg take in over 24 hours?

Question 6

A patient weighing 45kg is prescribed a dose of 3mg/kg. What dose should be given?

Question 7

A patient is prescribed to take 100mg of thiamine. Thiamine is available in 50mg tablets. How many tablets should be taken?

Question 8

Over a 24-hour period, Lee's fluid inputs are 700ml, 130ml, 480ml, 175ml and 50ml. His fluid outputs are 500ml, 350ml, 280ml, 435ml and 85ml. What is his total fluid input and output?

Question 9

A patient has an 80mg prescription of a drug that is available in a 1 in 100 solution. What volume of the solution should you give?

Question 10

What infusion rate (in millilitres per hour) would be required to deliver 600ml of a fluid over 1 hours, 30 minutes?

Question 11

A patient is prescribed 400mg of a drug to be delivered over 2 hours. The drug is available with a stock dose of 10mg/5ml that is delivered at 20 drops per ml. What should the drip rate be set at?

Question 12

How much fluid will be required in the first 24 hours for a patient weighing 45kg who has 20% of his body covered with burns?

Solutions

Worked solutions to test F can be accessed at <u>*www.mathsfornurses.com/practicetestse-h*</u>

1. 14ml

2. 30ml

3. 11.7ml

4. 405ml

5. Between 1850ml and 2590ml

6. 135mg

7. 2

8. Input – 1535ml, Output – 1650ml

9. 8ml

10. 400ml/hour

11. 33 drops per minute

12. 3600ml

Practice Test G

Question 1

A patient is prescribed 75mg of a drug t.d.s. How much of the drug will she be given over 24 hours?

Question 2

How much fluid will be required in the first 24 hours for a patient weighing 53kg who has 8% of her body covered with burns?

Question 3

A patient is prescribed 400mg of a drug that is available in 100mg in 50ml ampoules. How much of the solution should be administered?

Question 4

A patient weighing 75kg is prescribed 5mg/kg of a drug that is available in 25mg/10ml solution. How much of the solution should be given?

Question 5

A patient is prescribed 60mg of a drug to be taken every 4 hours. How much of the drug will be given over 24-hours?

Question 6

A patient is prescribed 16mg risperidone. The drug is available with a stock dose of 4mg/5ml. How much of the solution should be administered?

Question 7

Here is the fluid balance chart for a patient's fluid input and output over a 24-hour period.

| TIME | INPUT | | | | | OUTPUT | | |
	Oral Input	Volume	IV Input	Volume	Running Total	Urine	Other	Running Total
00:00								
01:00								
02:00								
03:00								
04:00						150ml		
05:00								
06:00								
07:00	Tea	100ml				200ml		
08:00								
09:00			0.9% Saline	500ml				
10:00							500ml	
11:00								
12:00	Water	100ml						
13:00						300ml		
14:00			0.9% Saline	650ml				
15:00								
16:00								
17:00							450ml	
18:00	Water	300ml						
19:00						200ml		
20:00								
21:00	Water	75ml						
22:00								
23:00								
Total								

Work out his total fluid input and output.

Question 8

Blood is delivered at 15 drips per ml. How long will it take to deliver 350mg of blood if the drip rate is set to 50 drips per minute?

Question 9

A patient weighing 18kg is prescribed a dose of 1.5mg/kg. What dose should be given?

Question 10

A patient is prescribed 75mg of a drug to be delivered over a period of 8 hours. The drug is available with a stock dose of 1mg/25ml that is delivered at 20 drops per ml. What should the drip rate be set at?

Question 11

A patient is prescribed 8mg of ramelteon to help with their sleep. How many 8mg tablets should the patient be given?

Question 12

A drug is available as a 5mg vial that has a displacement value of 0.1ml and needs to be made up as a solution containing 5mg in 10ml. How much fluid would you need to add to the solution?

Solutions

Worked solutions to test G can be accessed at www.mathsfornurses.com/practicetestse-h

1. 225mg

2. 1696ml

3. 200ml

4. 150ml

5. 360mg

6. 20ml

7. Input – 1725ml, Output – 1800ml

8. 1 hour, 45 minutes

9. 27mg

10. 78 drops per minute

11. 1

12. 9.9ml

Practice Test H

Question 1

How much fluid will be required in the first 24 hours for a patient weighing 68kg who has 28% of her body covered with burns?

Question 2

15mg of a drug is prescribed. The drug is available in 25mg tablets. If you were to crush one tablet and dissolve it in 10ml of water, what volume of the solution would you give to the patient?

Question 3

A patient is prescribed 10,000 International Units of dalteparin, which is available in 2,500 International Units in 0.2ml ampoules. How much of the solution should be administered to the patient?

Question 4

A patient is prescribed 45mg of codeine. How many codeine 15mg tablets should they be given?

Question 5

A patient is given a prescription for 150mg of cotrimoxazole. Cotrimoxazole is available in a solution with 25mg in 10ml. How much of the solution should be administered?

Question 6

A syringe with stroke length 60mm needs to be delivered over 4 hours. What rate should the syringe be set to in mm per hour?

Question 7

How much fluid should a child weighing 25kg take in over 24 hours?

Question 8

Over a 24-hour period, Isabelle's fluid inputs are 325ml, 280ml, 470ml, 100ml and 245ml. Her fluid outputs are 1200ml, 250ml, 35ml, and 80ml. Work out her total input and output for the day.

Question 9

What drip rate should you set to administer 1200ml of a fluid that is delivered at 20 drops per ml over a 12-hour period?

Question 10

A patient in prescribed 150mg of a drug that is available in 50mg in 30ml ampoules. How much of the solution should be administered?

Question 11

A patient is prescribed 85mg of a drug to be taken every 3 hours for 12 hours. How much of the drug will be given in total?

Question 12

A patient weighing 24kg is prescribed 0.8mg/kg of a drug that is available in a 1 in 500 solution. How much of the solution should be administered?

Solutions

Worked solutions to test H can be accessed at <u>www.mathsfornurses.com/practicetestse-h</u>

1. 7616ml

2. 6ml

3. 0.8ml

4. 3

5. 60ml

6. 15mm/hour

7. 1600ml

8. Input – 1420ml, Output – 1565ml

9. 33 drops per minute

10. 90ml

11. 340mg

12. 9.6ml

Printed in Great Britain
by Amazon